Visual Field Testing with the Humphrey Field Analyzer

A Text and Clinical Atlas

Second Edition

Visual Field Testing with the Humphrey Field Analyzer

A Text and Clinical Atlas

Second Edition

Neil T. Choplin, MD
Russell P. Edwards, MD

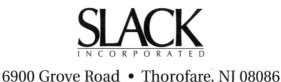

6900 Grove Road • Thorofare, NJ 08086

Publisher: John H. Bond
Editorial Director: Amy E. Drummond
Associate Editor: Jennifer L. Stewart

Choplin, Neil T.
    Visual Field Testing with the Humphrey Field Analyzer -- 2nd ed./Neil T. Choplin, Russell P. Edwards
        p. cm.
    Includes bibliographical references and index.
    ISBN 1-55642-389-6 (alk. paper)
    1. Perimetry. 2. Visual fields.
    [DNLM: 1. Perimetry--methods. 2. Perimetry--instrumentation.
3 Visual fields.   WW 145 C549v 1999]
RE79.P4C46   1999
617.7' 15--dc21
DNLM/DLC
for Library of Congress   99-26556
                                                                                             CIP

Published by: SLACK Incorporated
                 6900 Grove Road
                 Thorofare, NJ 08086-9447 USA
                 Telephone: 856-848-1000
                 Fax: 856-853-5991
                 World Wide Web: http://www.slackinc.com

Contact SLACK Incorporated for more information about other books in this field or about the availability of our books from distributors outside the United States.

Last digit is print number: 10 9 8 7 6 5 4 3 2 1

Dedication

To our residents and students who taught us much;
our families, who patiently saw us through this project;
and to the memory of Lillian A. Choplin.

Contents

Expanded Contents

Acknowledgments

The authors gratefully acknowledge the support, guidance, and help from the following people: George L. Spaeth, MD, who made Dr. Choplin the "field fellow"; Ray Sabatino and Tom Farrell, MD, who introduced Dr. Choplin to the Humphrey Field Analyzer; Rick Torney, who introduced us to the Humphrey Instruments Company and the field analyzer product managers over the years; MeeMee Wong, June Renne, Shareef Mahdavi, and Tom Chedwick, whose willingness to share material and answer questions has taught us much about the machine. Dr. Mike Patella from Humphrey Instruments has been a tremendous resource over the years in furthering our understanding of the workings of the instruments. We are also grateful to John Bond and Amy Drummond from SLACK Incorporated, who have helped and guided us through the preparation of the text.

Contributing Authors

Boel Bengtsson, PhD
Malmö University Hospital
Lunds University
Malmö, Sweden

Neil T. Choplin, MD
Clinical Associate Professor of Surgery
Uniformed Services University of Health Sciences
Captain, Medical Corps, United States Navy
Chairman, Department of Ophthalmology
Director, Glaucoma Service
Naval Medical Center
San Diego, California

Russell P. Edwards, MD
Captain, Medical Corps, United States Navy
Assistant Chairman, Department of Ophthalmology
Director, Neuro-Ophthalmology Service
Naval Medical Center
San Diego, California

Anders Heijl, MD, PhD
Professor and Chairman
Department of Ophthalmology
Malmö University Hospital
Lunds University
Malmö, Sweden

Pamela A. Sample, PhD
Associate Professor of Ophthalmology
Director of the Visual Function Laboratory
University of California, San Diego
La Jolla, California

Robert N. Weinreb, MD
Professor and Vice Chair of Ophthalmology
Glaucoma Center and Research Laboratories
University of California, San Diego
La Jolla, California

Foreword to the First Edition

Visual field examination is at the heart of the care of many patients with ocular and neurological diseases. After all, for many of these patients one of the primary goals of treatment is preservation of visual function.

Of all the tests of visual function, the measurements of acuity and field are unquestionably the most useful to the physician in directing diagnosis and management. This monograph deals with one of these characteristics from the point of view of two highly knowledgeable practitioners. The reader will find the material presented concisely and understandably, in a way that will help him or her in the daily management of patients. Automated computer perimetry permits the most standardized possible evaluation of the visual field. Software advances provide the physician with suggestions as to whether the field is "normal," or "abnormal," whether the defects found are of clinical significance, whether the field is stable or changing, as well as many other interpretive considerations, such as whether the visual field is reliable. These entries on the printed sheet of visual field results take on the appearance of scientific fact, and busy practitioners, who are always looking for certainty and who are pressed for time, are quick to utilize such interpretations in their diagnosis and management of patients. It is all too easy to forget that these software evaluations are themselves soft and demand thoughtful interpretation in order for them to be utilized in a way that is in fact going to be in the patient's best interest.

Drs. Choplin and Edwards' monograph leads the reader through the thought processes that are involved in deciding what type of visual field examination to choose and how to interpret the results in a way that will provide the most useful clinical information. Enough theory is included to permit a thorough understanding of the principles that underlie the hardware methodologies and software interpretations.

Computerized perimetry is now unquestionably the standard by which other perimetric evaluations are judged. The Humphrey computerized perimeter is now widely distributed. Information from normal individuals and glaucoma patients has been accumulated and has allowed for the development of clinically useful software. Ophthalmologists utilizing the Humphrey instrument will find this monograph by Choplin and Edwards very helpful.

—George L. Spaeth, MD

Preface to the First Edition

"Humphrey field un-interpretable, get a Goldmann." This statement greeted me in more than one patient record upon my arrival at the Navy Hospital in San Diego in 1985. Inside the medical record would be a full-page graytone printout with no other information, followed by the aforementioned Goldmann field. The Humphrey Field Analyzer was sitting in a corner of the visual field area, with its dust cover in place, waiting for someone to figure out what to do with it, other than use it for a punch bowl.

My experience with automated perimetry began with the Octopus 201. There were three of them at the Wills Eye Hospital in Philadelphia, and they turned out a visual field printout unlike anything I had ever seen before. My first assignment as a glaucoma fellow was to interpret the visual fields that were done in the Glaucoma Service Diagnostic Laboratory and send written reports to the referring physicians. A stack of such fields awaited me when I reported for my first day on the service. Looking at the threshold printouts, I asked, "Where is the book that explains what these numbers mean?" There was no book, no manual, no user's guide. Just tables of numbers representing the visual field. I hit the library. Nothing. A literature search turned up some of the original research done in Switzerland by the people who developed the Octopus perimeter (some of whom are listed in the *Suggested Reading* at the end of this book). A few weeks of looking at the printouts, coupled with repeated readings of the original papers and discussions with people familiar with automated perimetry, finally brought to me a rudimentary understanding of some of the principles of automated perimetry. I set out to write a guideline to visual field interpretation, not so much for others but to cement my own understanding. The resulting monograph was put together by Cilco (then the distributor of the Octopus perimeter) and had limited distribution.

Shortly after the beginning of my fellowship in 1984, the general ophthalmology service at Wills Eye Hospital received a Humphrey Field Analyzer for evaluation. As the designated "field fellow," I was asked to "go study it." The Humphrey came with something I couldn't find with the Octopus—a user's manual! I read it. More than once. Automated perimetry began to make more sense. Contained within the manual was a conversion table for decibels to apostilbs. I looked at the numbers, took out a calculator, and figured out how to convert from one to the other. It dawned on me, after playing with the numbers, that the decibel scale represented attenuation of the maximum available stimulus. I excitedly reported my discovery to Dr. Spaeth, who replied, "Of course." Together with the chief of the general ophthalmology service, we began a systematic study of the Humphrey, comparing it to the Octopus by testing patients known to have abnormal visual fields. The "new kid on the block" measured up pretty well to the "gold standard" for automated perimetry, which has been borne out by the success of the instrument.

Armed with this elementary knowledge of automated perimetry and my early experience with the Humphrey Field Analyzer, I arrived in San Diego and realized I had to convert the Department of Ophthalmology into the ways of the state of the art. This book represents the results of the conversion process. Most of the little tricks and pearls contained in the following chapters are things I learned the hard way. My co-author, Russ Edwards, having both an interest in neuro-ophthalmology and a broad knowledge base in the ways of computers, proved to be a most capable traveling companion on the road to construction of a usable perimetry system. We continually challenge each other with interesting cases and pop into each others' offices with a printout in hand (check this out!). We now have 30 years of experience with the Humphrey Field Analyzer between us and have enjoyed sharing our experiences through courses at the annual meeting of the American Academy of Ophthalmology and the Joint Commission for Allied Health Personnel in Ophthalmology. This book represents an expansion of the courses we teach together at those meetings. It includes tricks and bits of knowledge we learned from other users of the machine who attended our course. I hope readers of this text will benefit from our experiences, find useful information for organizing a perimetry system, make good use of what the machine has to offer, and make the perimetry experience better for their patients.

Disclaimer

Although Dr. Edwards and I are active duty members of the Medical Corps, United States Navy, this book is not being written as part of our official duties. This book is written about the Humphrey Field Analyzer because it is the machine that we use. Decisions to purchase the machine were made prior to my arrival in 1984. We have stayed with the Humphrey Field Analyzer because we have an extensive collection of patient data, we understand how the machine works and what can be done with it, and have not had any reason to switch to any other perimeter. This book, however, is not intended to be a commercial endorsement of the Humphrey Field Analyzer. Neither of us has any proprietary interest in the company or the product, and this work was not sponsored in any way by the company. Many other perimeters are on the market that have the same capabilities as the Humphrey instrument and would serve the purposes of most clinicians. We assume that the reader of this book is reading it for the same reason that we wrote it: because he or she is a user of the instrument and would like to maximize his or her understanding of how it can be used to provide quality care to patients. The views and opinions expressed in this work are ours alone and are not intended to be construed as official opinions of the Department of the Navy or of the Department of Defense.

—Neil T. Choplin, MD

Preface to the Second Edition

At the time the first edition of this text was published, the Humphrey Field Analyzer II had just been released. The 700 series is now available on the market. This edition has been revised to include material pertaining to the new series of perimeters as well as the software and hardware advances that have been made. Included are new discussions of short-wavelength automated perimetry (SWAP), the Swedish Interactive Thresholding Algorithm (SITA), and the hardware changes that distinguish the Humphrey Field Analyzer II from its older relatives. We have also expanded the discussions of managing a visual field testing system to cover most possibilities. However, we have not eliminated any of the material pertinent to the older models so that hopefully this text will be useful to old and new users alike, whichever model perimeter they may use. As with the first edition, the authors invite readers to communicate with us and let us know what they find useful in their practices for inclusion in future editions.

—Neil T. Choplin, MD
—Russell P. Edwards, MD

Introduction

The Humphrey Field Analyzer represents one of many remarkable eye care instruments developed by Humphrey Instruments of San Leandro, Calif. The company was founded by William Humphrey, PhD, in 1971 and had its start with an automated refraction system developed by Dr. Humphrey and Louis Alvarez, PhD, a Nobel laureate in physics. The system performed subjective refractions without the use of conventional lenses and without a machine in front of the patient's face. The Vision Analyzer, as the system was called, was marketed in 1977. The analyzer was an overnight success and propelled the company into a growth mode of new product development. One year later, the company introduced an instrument for automatically neutralizing spectacle lenses.

Automated static perimetry reached into clinical practice with the Octopus perimeters in the late 1970s. The original Octopus 201 perimeter was room-sized and very expensive, costing in excess of $100,000. The relatively unknown technology and high cost of the system kept automated perimetry in the "ivory tower." Recognizing the advantages of automated static threshold perimetry and seeing a large market in the eye care world outside of academic medicine, Humphrey Instruments began development of a perimeter for the masses. The first prototypes of the Humphrey Field Analyzer were displayed at the American Academy of Ophthalmology meeting in 1982. Later that year, clinical technique development was begun by Anders Heijl, MD, and Michael Patella, OD, culminating in the completion of a clinical prototype in August 1983. In November 1983, 10 prototype clinical units were sent to glaucoma centers for beta site testing. Production unit delivery began in February of 1984. Because of its relatively small size and low cost, the machine became very popular.

The early models of the Humphrey Field Analyzer used the concept of an individualized island of vision for determining visual field abnormalities. Each eye being tested would have expected normal values calculated based upon a few initial test points, and the results compared to those expected values. Although this was a good way to identify focal loss within the visual field, there was no way of telling whether or not the overall level of the island of vision was normal. Octopus had age-corrected normals right from the beginning, and patients were compared to a normal database. Desire for age-corrected normals led to the development of STATPAC, first released for sale in November 1986 after two and a half years in development.

Improvements in hardware and software have continued. STATPAC 2 was released in 1989, FASTPAC in 1991, and blue-yellow testing capability became available in November 1993. The Humphrey Field Analyzer has become representative of the state of the art in automated static perimetry with over 35,000 instruments sold worldwide as of the date of this book. The Humphrey Field Analyzer II was introduced in 1995 and included (as an option) short-wavelength automated perimetry (blue-yellow, SWAP). A new, shorter method for performing full threshold testing was introduced in 1997: SITA (Swedish Interactive Thresholding Algorithm).

This book is about automated perimetry and the Humphrey Field Analyzer. It deals with many aspects of perimetry, from the hardware and software of the machine to organization of a perimetry system and the test area. It also deals with decision making: what test to do, how to do it, and how to run a test in such a manner as to reduce the possibility of obtaining unreliable and useless information. Suggestions for making the machine operator's job easier and for helping the patient "survive" the test are also given. Some of the material may be found in more than one chapter. Although we prefer to avoid redundancy, we felt it better to discuss some items in context rather than force the reader to jump from place to place. Wherever possible, all references to items under discussion are cited. The illustrations are not repeated in different places, therefore if an illustration can be used to highlight a point in a different chapter, the reader will be referred to it.

Two appendices are provided at the end of the text. Appendix A allows the reader to locate examples of visual field defects occurring in different diseases of the visual system within the book. The examples contained in this book are not intended to be inclusive of all types of visual field defects that are possible in a particular disease nor of all diseases affecting the visual field. Appendix B is a listing of visual fields by the main finding in the book so that the reader can see a representative example of a particular type of field defect. Again, this text is not intended to be inclusive of all possible visual field abnormalities, but is intended to display how the Humphrey Field Analyzer portrays a particular defect.

In 14 years of Humphrey Field Analyzer use, we have probably encountered most of the pitfalls and obstacles to satisfactory visual field testing. We hope that the reader will benefit from the mistakes we have seen and our proposed solutions to avoiding or minimizing them. The reader should bear in mind that what is contained in this book is the result of what we have found to work for us. Feel free to adopt or adapt anything in this book, from ordering forms to patient instruction sheets. We would be pleased to hear how your system works for you and how it differs from the one we describe here.

You may notice that the appearance of the visual field printouts in this book are slightly different from the way yours may look. We use a LaserJet IIIp printer connected to the RS232C port on the back of the machine. This printer is available from Humphrey, and the software to run the printer is part of the most recent versions of the operating software. Check with the company to see if any other laser printer will work. You will have to check your owner's manual to see if your version is compatible with the laser printer, or check with your service representative. The laser printer gives the printout a slightly different look from the built-in dot matrix printer. Since single sheets are printed instead of a continuous printout, any of the "change over time" printouts are limited to three fields per page. The illustrations have been cut and pasted to give the appearance of a continuous printout. Most printouts have been trimmed but otherwise look as they do when they come out of the machine. An occasional printout has been "rearranged" for illustrative purposes and will not come out of the machine as pictured. No data has been altered in any way, and the examples provided in the text are real clinical examples of visual fields from the patients under our care.

This book is not intended to be a substitute for the owner's manual. The operator instructions provided with the field analyzer are quite good and complete. It was not our intention to rewrite the owner's manual but rather to show the reader some of the ways the material contained in the manual can be adapted to a particular clinical situation. Our suggestions do not apply to all circumstances, and we certainly would not like to see everything done our way. We present what we have found useful and trust that the reader will take away what will be useful to him or her. Read the owner's manual (as we have), make sure the technicians read the manual, and keep it handy for reference. We hope this work will be a good supplement to what you already know.

—Neil T. Choplin, MD
—Russell P. Edwards, MD

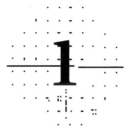

Introduction to Automated Perimetry

The Visual Field

The visual field is that portion of space which is visible to an individual at any given moment. Many diseases and conditions affecting the visual system manifest themselves through changes in the visual field, and determining the extent of the visual field is an important aspect of the diagnosis and management of those conditions. Although visual space is normally perceived with both eyes, for most purposes the visual field of each eye of an individual is measured separately. Once the field has been defined for each eye, the two visual fields can be compared to each other for asymmetry, compared to a "normal" reference base for abnormality, and examined together to look for patterns suggestive of different conditions.

Perimetry is the science of measuring ("-metry") the peripheral ("peri-") vision in order to determine the visual field. Methods employed in perimetry have evolved and adapted to advances in technology, particularly electronics and computer science. Modern visual field testing as such is much more than a determination of the limits of visual space—modern techniques allow for examination of the entire visual field, including the central field, and help to broaden our understanding of the conditions we are testing.

The Island of Vision

In 1927, Traquair likened the visual field of an individual eye to an "island of vision in a sea of blindness" (see Duke-Elder S. in *Suggested Reading*). This island (or hill) of vision analogy serves as the model for visual field testing. Determination of the island of vision is a matter of drawing a map of the island for the eye(s) being tested. Figure 1-1 is a depiction of the island of vision. Regardless of its extent or shape, an important aspect of the analogy is that the island of vision is a three-dimensional structure. For the purposes of most "maps," the fovea is the visual field point with the X and Y coordinates corresponding to 0, 0. The location of the other visual field points can be expressed as an X, Y pair with respect to fixation. The unit used for the X and Y axes is degrees from fixation. The Z axis represents the height of the island of vision at the point X, Y and corresponds to the sensitivity of the retina at that point. The greater the sensitivity at any point, the greater the height of the island of vision. The fovea in the normal visual field is the "peak" of the island, since it has the greatest sensitivity.

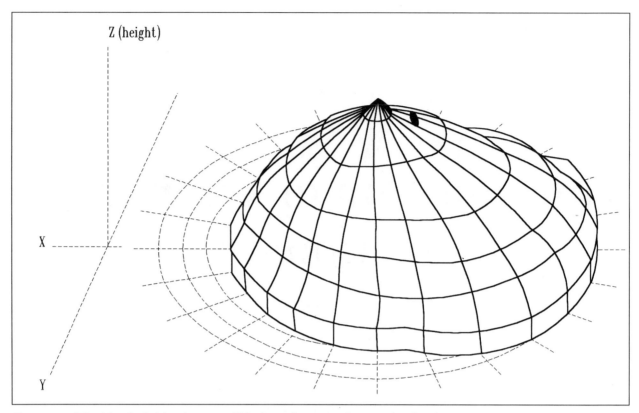

Figure 1-1. "The island of vision in a sea of blindness." Drawing by Lynn R. Choplin.

Mapping the Island of Vision

With the island of vision analogy, perimetry becomes a matter of drawing the map of the island of vision. The method used to draw the map is not important as long as the map obtained is accurate (ie, is a true representation of the island for the eye being tested and the information is presented in such a way as to be clinically useful. The earliest testing methods involved defining the limits of visual space by moving objects from areas of non-seeing toward the center, with the patient indicating in some manner when the object was seen. The technique of testing the visual field by moving objects of fixed size and intensity is known as *kinetic perimetry* and is the technique employed when using the tangent screen or the Goldmann perimeter. For each test object of fixed size and intensity (corresponding to a fixed height along the island), the boundary of the island is determined at that height. The area surrounded by this boundary is known as an *isopter*, and each isopter is analogous to a horizontal slice through the island of vision. Areas of the island inside each isopter boundary would be expected to have equal or greater sensitivity to the points at the boundary. An area within a given isopter showing less than expected sensitivity is known as a *scotoma*. Determining multiple isopters and then stacking them one on top of the other gives the two-dimensional picture of the island of vision that is familiar to most clinicians. The map of a normal island of vision as determined by isopter perimetry is shown in Figure 1-2, bottom. This is the view of the island of vision that can be obtained by hovering directly over the island and viewing it from above.

The island of vision can also be determined by measuring the sensitivity of the retina at each X, Y point, establishing the height. This can be accomplished by varying the intensity of a test object of fixed size and location until the appropriate response has been elicited to define the sensitivity; the values obtained are considered to be "threshold" measurements. Since the test location is held stationary to determine threshold, this type of perimetric testing is known as *static perimetry*. The Tubinger perimeter performed static perimetry along individual meridia of the island of vision, giving rise to the term *profile perimetry*. Combining these multiple vertical slices taken through various meridia by static techniques, like stacking the horizontal cuts

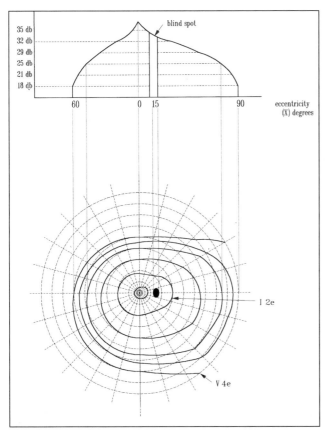

Figure 1-2. Views of the island of vision. Top: A vertical slice through the 0° to 180° meridian, yielding a profile of the island as viewed from the side. Bottom: Horizontal slices through the island of vision, giving the familiar isopter plot. This is the view of the island from the top (adapted from Harrington DO. *The Visual Fields.* 4th ed. St. Louis, Mo: CV Mosby Publishers; 1976. Drawing by Lynn R. Choplin).

obtained by kinetic perimetry, yields a graphical representation of the three-dimensional island of vision. Figure 1-2, top, is a vertical slice through the island of vision. The blind spot appears to the right of the peak, located as expected at 15° temporal to fixation. This view of the island is obtained by viewing it from the side or from "sea" level.

Rationale for Automation in Perimetry

The performance of accurate perimetry is a difficult task. Administering a visual field test by Goldmann perimetry in a glaucoma patient, for example, requires a combination of kinetic (to define isopter boundaries) and static (to find nasal steps and paracentral defects) techniques, taking 20 to 30 minutes per eye. Setting up the machine, determining the correct isopters, preparing the patient, monitoring fixation, moving and adjusting the stimulus projector, presenting the stimuli for static presentations, recording the patient's responses, repeating for the sufficient number of isopters to draw a good map, and preparing the "map" are exacting tasks. Static perimetry and the determination of threshold is particularly difficult due to the large number of stimulus presentations that may be required to accurately determine the retinal sensitivity at all of the test points. In addition, it may be difficult for a human examiner to avoid introducing bias into an otherwise subjective examination, thereby reducing the accuracy of the examination. An examiner may wish, consciously or unconsciously, for an examination to be "normal" and may fail to detect defects; similarly, nonexistent "defects" may be discovered if the examiner wishes them to be present. Likewise, follow-up examinations become subject to inaccuracies, particularly if performed by different examiners, due to variations in technique as well as other "human" factors. Results of such examinations are dependent upon the interaction between the examiner (technician) and the patient and may be influenced by that interaction in the absence of any visual field abnormalities.

Automated visual field testing systems have been developed over the past 15 to 20 years in an attempt to eliminate some of the above problems. Computer-controlled test procedures can be standardized and are not subject to examiner bias. Selection of test points (once the clinician has chosen the area to be examined), stimulus intensity values and how they are varied, order of presentation of stimuli to test points, recording of patient responses, retesting of missed points, monitoring of fixation, performance of "catch trials" as measures of reliability, and printouts of results are all functions easily adapted to machines. In addition, visual field data can be manipulated by the computer into various formats that ease interpretation for the clinician, can be stored, compared to known normals, and recalled at the time of follow-up procedures for evaluation with regard to change. Finally, automation has allowed a transition from manually controlled (ie, by the technician) kinetic perimetry to computer-controlled static threshold perimetry, which has been shown to be capable of detecting loss (particularly centrally) earlier than the older techniques.

Various machine designs have evolved since the advent of perimetry automation. All machines perform static perimetry in one form or another, with most having the capability of determining threshold at the points tested. Some have the capacity to perform automated kinetic perimetry and define isopters. Stimulus presentation methods vary, ranging from a moving projector capable of testing any point within the bowl, fixed light emitting diodes with limited flexibility for testing outside of established patterns, to machines with moving fixation targets capable of testing any point in the field by moving the eye to the target. Some machines use the computer solely to control the test, while other machines utilize either an internal or external computer for data storage and manipulation.

The Humphrey Field Analyzer is an automated static threshold perimeter that has gained wide acceptance and usage throughout the world. Although the machine performs most of the actual testing, it is just one part of the overall visual field system. The clinician, technician, and patient are all integral parts of the system necessary for the generation of an accurate visual field map. All parts of the system must work optimally to achieve the desired result.

Chapter 3 describes one type of visual field system organization. The clinician must know what information is being sought from the visual field test so that the most appropriate examination and test parameters can be selected (described in Chapter 4), and the perimetrist must know the "nuts and bolts" of the machine (Chapter 2) and how to properly set-up and administer the test (Chapter 4). Finally, the patient must be properly prepared to take the test in order to perform optimally (Chapter 4). Automated perimetry presents visual field information in a way that may not be familiar to some clinicians, therefore proper interpretation of the results is essential if the system is to have any worth. Interpretation of automated visual fields as performed by the Humphrey Field Analyzer will be discussed in Chapter 5.

Definition of Terms Used in Automated Perimetry

Static perimetry requires the patient to make a response to a projected stimulus of fixed size, location, and duration of presentation at a given intensity level. In order to understand what static perimetry is measuring, it is necessary to understand the terms and units used to express the results.

THRESHOLD

The results of a visual field test may be presented in many different formats, depending upon the machine used and the available software. Common to all formats (in one form or another) is the concept of threshold. Even in kinetic perimetry, the drawn boundary of an isopter is a threshold measurement, delineating areas capable of seeing a target (inside the line) from areas that cannot.

When a stimulus is projected against a background, the patient has only two possible responses: push the response button (implying that the stimulus was seen) or do not push the response button (implying that the stimulus was not seen). Because of the possibility of false responses, the response or lack of a response is just an implication, not actual proof, that the light was seen or not seen. For a stimulus of fixed size and location, there is a certain probability that it will be seen, which is dependent upon its intensity. This probability can be plotted against the stimulus intensity, giving a frequency of seeing, or probability of perception, curve. One such hypothetical curve is shown in Figure 1-3.

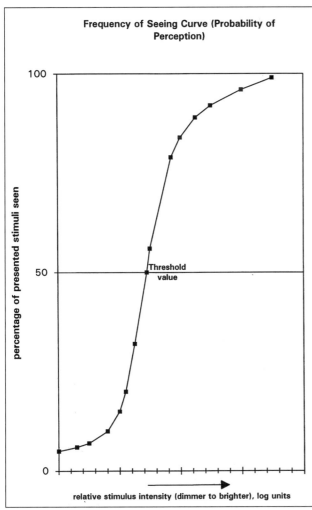

Frequency of Seeing Curve (Probability of Perception)

y-axis: percentage of presented stimuli seen (0, 50, 100)

Threshold value

x-axis: relative stimulus intensity (dimmer to brighter), log units

Figure 1-3. Probability of seeing a stimulus as a function of its intensity: the frequency of seeing or probability of perception curve.

For any given stimulus at a visual field point, there is a certain probability that a response will be elicited, proportional to its intensity. Dim stimuli approach (but never reach) 0% probability of eliciting a response, and bright lights approach (but never reach) 100% probability. A very bright light projected into the central portion of the visual field has a very high probability of being seen, while a dim light projected into the far periphery has a very small chance of being seen and eliciting a response. However, human beings are not perfect test subjects, and there is a certain amount of inaccuracy built into their ability to respond in a test situation. If told to push a button when presented with a light, even a blind person may on occasion think a light was seen when a dim light is presented to the periphery of the field. Similarly, a bright light projected onto the fovea of a young healthy adult may on occasion fail to elicit a response. Lights with low probabilities of perception will on occasion elicit a response, and those with a high probability of perception will on occasion fail to do so. These considerations give rise to the definition of threshold (corresponding to the height of the island of vision at the test point). Threshold for a given point is defined as that stimulus intensity (for an object of fixed size and duration of presentation) that has a 50% probability of being seen. One important consideration based on this definition is that each time threshold is determined, it is possible to obtain a different answer. In fact, this variability, known as *fluctuation*, is measurable in the normal population and has clinical significance. Fluctuation is discussed in greater detail in Chapters 5 and 6.

Determination of Threshold

It would be impractical to test each point in the field with thousands of stimuli of varying intensity to find the one that is seen 50% of the time. Fortunately, an algorithm exists that has an accuracy of ± one decibel (decibel [dB], is a measure of relative light intensity and will be discussed later in this chapter) 99% of

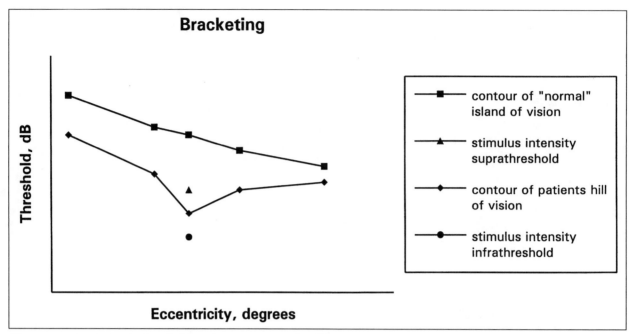

Figure 1-4. Bracketing in threshold testing. Some stimuli will be brighter than threshold and some will be dimmer during the process of determining threshold.

the time. This algorithm varies the intensity of the presented stimuli according to the patient's response to the previous stimulus. The concepts involved are:

Bracketing

During determination of threshold at each point in the test grid, stimulus intensities will vary in such a way that some will be suprathreshold (brighter than necessary to elicit a response most of the time) and some will be infrathreshold (too dim to elicit a response most of the time). This is illustrated in Figure 1-4. Threshold is thus "bracketed" by the test stimuli as the examination proceeds.

Double Crossing of Threshold

Unless using a nonstandard test strategy, such as FASTPAC or SITA (Swedish Interactive Thresholding Algorithm), stimulus intensities are varied during the test according to the patient's responses in such a manner that threshold will be crossed twice. This is illustrated in Figure 1-5. In this example, the first stimulus presented at point P is seen (open circle, labeled "1"), and the patient pushes the response button. The machine then tests that point again with a dimmer stimulus, turning down the intensity by four decibels. Stimulus 2 was also seen, indicated by the open circle. This process continues until the stimulus is too dim to elicit a response (stimulus 3: lack of response indicated by closed circle), that is, the intensity is now below threshold and threshold has been crossed for the first time. The machine now makes the stimuli brighter in two-decibel steps until the patient pushes the button, indicating the second crossing of threshold (stimulus 4 was not seen, stimulus 5 was). Since the step size was two decibels, threshold is the value that lies between the intensity values of the last two stimuli. Obviously, if the first stimulus presented to the point was not seen, the machine will make the stimuli brighter in four-decibel steps until threshold is crossed and then dimmer in two-decibel steps until the second crossing. On the average, it takes five stimulus presentations at each point to determine threshold. The Humphrey Field Analyzer always begins testing with a stimulus six decibels brighter than expected normal, except when using the "fast" threshold strategy, as explained in Chapter 2.

Random Stimulus Presentations

If the machine continually presented stimuli to one point in the field until threshold was determined, the patient would quickly learn where the next stimulus would be. Therefore, the machine tests points randomly during the course of the test, with the computer keeping track of the prior responses at each point, vary-

Figure 1-5. The algorithm used for threshold determination at a visual field point, P. Open circles indicate patient response to stimulus, filled circles indicate no response to stimulus. Down arrow indicates stimuli decreasing in four-decibel steps, up arrow indicates stimuli increasing in two-decibel steps. Numbers indicate order of stimulus presentation.

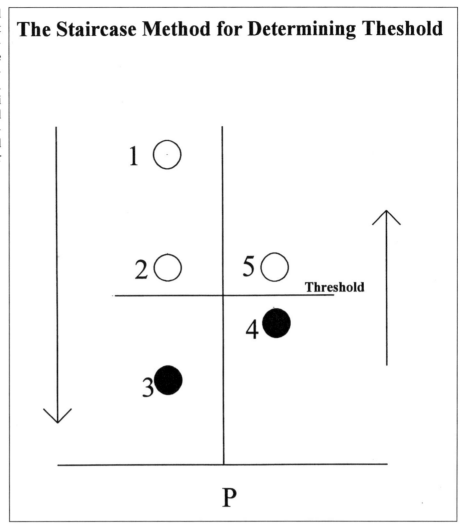

ing the next stimulus intensity accordingly. The point being tested will flash on the CRT (cathode ray tube) display, and the threshold number will appear when the determination is complete.

Nonstandard Threshold Algorithms

Because of the large amount of time needed to generate threshold data for all of the test points in a full threshold test, newer algorithms have been developed to speed up the test procedures. FASTPAC uses a three-decibel step and crosses threshold once, saving between 25% to 40% of test time. Since the final step is three decibels instead of two, there is more variability in repeated measures of threshold, which could have clinical significance if a clinician places value on measurement of fluctuation (see Chapter 5). SITA, (see Chapter 9), relies heavily upon a large database of normal and abnormal visual fields to estimate threshold values based on the pattern of patient responses during the test. It may save more than 50% of test time. Experience with this algorithm has been minimal as of the date of this publication, but it appears promising as a means of speeding up a test without sacrificing accuracy.

Normal Threshold Values

Figure 1-6 illustrates the two main influences on normal threshold values (ie, location in the field and age). Note that the most sensitive point in the field, as expected, is the fovea, corresponding to 0° of eccentricity. Sensitivity then decreases as the points move away from the center, indicated by lower threshold values. The slope of the decrease is known from studies of the normal population and is not linear, that is the slope constantly changes from point to point. As a rough approximation, however, the sensitivity of the visu-

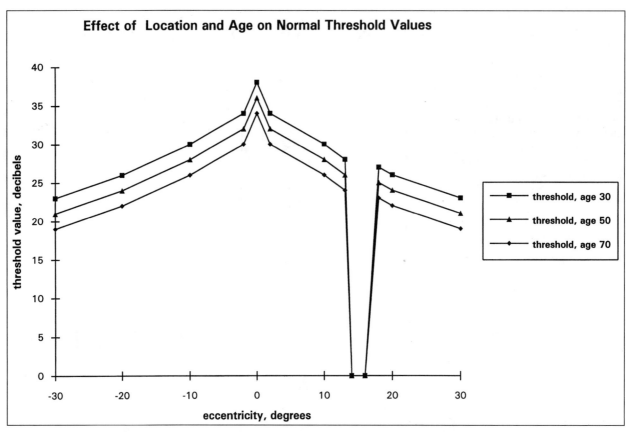

Figure 1-6. Factors determining normal threshold values.

al field outside of the macula (beyond 5° of eccentricity) decreases about 0.3 dB for each degree of eccentricity. This drop-off in sensitivity from the center toward the periphery is what gives the island of vision its characteristic shape. Sensitivity also decreases with age, as indicated by the lower curves in Figure 1-6. The decrease is uniform across the field and is on the magnitude of 0.6 to one decibel per point for each decade of life. As will be discussed later, because of the age-related change in threshold, it is important to make sure the patient's birth date is correctly entered into the machine if the results are to be compared to an age-related normal population.

Units Used to Express Threshold

A visual field test on the Humphrey Field Analyzer is performed by projecting lights into the bowl. The light reflects off of the bowl back toward the patient's eye. The intensity of light reflecting off of a surface is expressed in units of luminance, which is a measure of light density (ie, units of light per a unit of area). Different measurement systems have led to a great deal of confusion in terminology—candela per meter squared (NIT), foot-lambert, millilambert, and apostilb are all different units used for expressing luminance. The apostilb (abbreviated as asb) is the unit that is used most in static threshold perimetry. One apostilb can be thought of as the equivalent amount of light coming off of one square centimeter of solidifying platinum at 2040° Kelvin. Figure 1-7 shows the luminance values of some common objects. Noteworthy is the maximum stimulus intensity of the Humphrey Field Analyzer, which is roughly equivalent to the amount of light coming off of the full moon on a clear night. This value is 10,000 asb.

Although measured in apostilbs, it is not convenient to express threshold values in apostilbs. A printout of thresholds expressed in apostilbs would be difficult to read, since the sensitivity of the human visual system ranges from approximately one apostilb to more than 1,000,000 asb, a range of more than six log units. A printout would therefore have numbers ranging from single digits to five digits and would be messy. Fortunately, the expression of luminance values on a relative scale is convenient and appropriate to the way

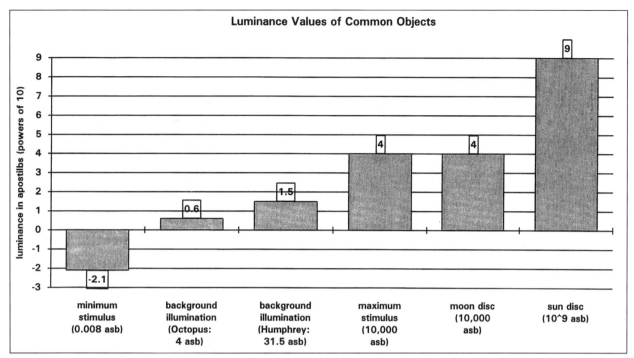

Figure 1-7. Luminance values of known objects.

the human visual system perceives changes in light intensity. A small change of one or a few apostilbs, particularly in the upper end of the range (ie, brighter stimuli), is not detectable. However, the human eye is capable of detecting a change (brighter or dimmer) if the stimulus is changed by a power of 10 or fraction thereof. Thus, it is convenient to express threshold values in terms of a relative logarithmic scale in which the stimulus intensities are varied by powers of 10. The scale used is the decibel scale, in which one decibel is equal to one-tenth of a log unit (power of 10). The decibel scale expresses threshold as a fraction of the maximum available stimulus intensity (ie, it measures how much the maximum available stimulus intensity was attenuated [dimmed] until threshold was determined using the above algorithm). It is important to realize that the apostilb value expressed by the decibel number is relative to the maximum available stimulus intensity on a particular instrument and will vary from one perimeter to another if the maximum available stimulus intensities are different. The Humphrey Field Analyzer changes the stimulus intensity by interposing filters of increasing density in front of the projector bulb in order to affect the desired attenuation.

To illustrate the relationship between light intensity expressed in apostilbs and decibels, assume the maximum available stimulus intensity is 10,000, or 10^4 asb, as is the case with the Humphrey Field Analyzer. If the brightest available stimulus was determined to be the threshold value at a point, it would be represented by 0 dB of attenuation. A "0" would appear on the printout of threshold values, indicating that to be the case (threshold values less than 0 [eg, the patient failed to respond to the maximum stimulus intensity] would be indicated by "< 0"). If the threshold value was recorded as "1," it would mean that the 10,000 asb maximum available stimulus was dimmed by 0.1 log units. The apostilb value of this stimulus would be $10^{4-0.1}$, or $10^{3.9}$, which equals 7943 asb. Similarly, attenuation of the maximum available stimulus by four decibels (indicated by a "4" on the value table printout) would mean that threshold was equal to $10^{4-0.1\times4}$, or $10^{3.6}$, which equals 3981 asb. Note that the decibel scale is linear (ie, changing in units), while the apostilb scale is not.

To convert decibel numbers to apostilb value, simply multiply the decibel number by 0.1 to convert to the power of 10, by which the 10^4 maximum stimulus is being attenuated; subtract that number from 4.0 to get the resultant power of 10, and raise 10 to that power. The formula is thus:

$$asb = 10^{4.0 - dB \times 0.1}$$

Table 1-1 relates decibels, apostilbs, and Goldmann equivalents. This information is useful if a visual field tested with a specific Goldmann target is required, as is sometimes specified by state disability examinations. The field can then be tested using the "single intensity" screening test, as discussed in Chapter 2, with the intensity set to the specified Goldmann equivalent.

The ability to convert decibels to apostilbs is not all that important and not something that needs to be done (unless trying to compare two fields that were performed on different machines with different maximum stimuli). What is important to realize is that as the decibel numbers increase on a value table printout, the maximum available stimulus intensity is being turned down by an increasing amount (larger number subtracted from four means a smaller resultant power of 10 and hence a dimmer stimulus). Threshold corresponding to a dimmer stimulus means greater retinal sensitivity. Thus, on a value table printout, which is the report of the patient's actual measured thresholds, larger decibel values correspond to better sensitivity, and smaller decibel numbers indicate loss of sensitivity. Determining the extent of loss and its clinical meaning will be discussed in many other areas of this text. The actual attenuation of the light intensity on the Humphrey Field Analyzer is accomplished by interposing filters of increasing density in front of the projector bulb.

TERMS USED TO DESCRIBE VISUAL FIELD ABNORMALITIES AND LOSS

Visual field loss means an alteration in the height and shape of the island of vision. Points in the field will show decreases in sensitivity from the levels they should have (alteration of height) and will not show the expected changes from neighboring points due to eccentricity (alteration of shape). Figure 1-8 illustrates common visual field defects as recorded by static threshold techniques on an automated perimeter. The top curve of the figure represents a profile of a "normal" island of vision for a person of a certain age. The middle curve is from a patient with a disease process that diffusely affects all points in the visual field. Note that the shape of the curve is the same as the "normal" island, but that all of the points manifest a uniform decrease in sensitivity. This is called *diffuse depression*, or "generalized reduction in sensitivity." If this field was mapped with isopter perimetry on a Goldmann perimeter, all of the isopters would appear smaller than they should, with the circumferences of the isopters moved toward the center of the plot. This is known as "constriction" of the visual field, and is thus analogous to diffuse depression as recorded on static threshold perimetry. Factors that influence the visual field to produce such diffuse loss of sensitivity will be discussed in subsequent chapters.

The lower curve in Figure 1-8 shows diffuse depression as well, but also shows additional loss centered around 20° nasally. This additional depression beyond any diffuse depression is known as *focal loss*, or as a *scotoma*. Webster's Dictionary defines a scotoma as "an area of pathologically diminished vision within the visual field," derived from the Latin word for dim sight and from the Greek word "skotos," or darkness. Since threshold information is quantitative, it is possible to determine the exact amount of sensitivity loss at each point by subtracting the patient's measured threshold value from that of the expected "normal" value. This is known as the defect depth and would be expressed in decibels. The larger the defect depth, the more pathological the field. The arrow in Figure 1-8 indicates the defect depth for the scotoma at 20° nasally. Since the visual field exhibits a combination of diffuse loss and focal loss, if one wanted to determine the extent of the focal loss only, it would be necessary to "correct" the island of vision for the diffuse loss by raising all of the threshold values by an amount equal to the average diffuse loss. Following such correction, any defects left over would represent focal loss. Techniques for performing such data manipulation will be discussed in Chapter 5.

Defects can be characterized by the magnitude of their depth—those between 5 and 9 dB from expected are "shallow," 10 to 19 dB may be considered "moderate," defects over 20 dB are "deep," and threshold less than the maximum available stimulus intensity is considered "absolute." It should be pointed out that the measurement of an absolute defects does not necessarily mean total loss of sensitivity—it only means that the machine was not capable of generating a stimulus bright enough to elicit a response.

Table 1-1

DECIBEL/APOSTILB/GOLDMANN EQUIVALENTS

Intensity dB	Asb	I	II	III	IV	V
			Actual Humphrey	Test Stimulus	Size	
0	10,000	III4e	IV4e	V4e		
1	7943	III4d	IV4d	V4d		
2	6310	III4c	III4c	V4c		
3	5012	III4b	IV4b	V4b		
4	3981	III4b	IV4b	V4b		
5	3162	II4e	III4e	IV4e	V4e	
6	2512	II4d	III4d	IV4d	V4d	
7	1995	II4c	III4c	III4c	V4c	
8	1585	II4b	III4b	IV4b	V4b	
9	1259	II4b	III4a	IV4a	V4a	
10	1000	I4e	II4e	III4e	IV4e	V4e
11	794	I4d	II4d	III4d	IV4d	V4d
12	631	I4c	II4c	III4c	IV4c	V4c
13	501	I4b	II4b	III4b	IV4b	V4b
14	398	I4a	II4a	III4a	IV4a	V4a
15	316	I3e	II3e	III3e	IV3e	V3e
16	251	I3d	II3d	III3d	IV3d	V3d
17	200	I3c	II3c	III3c	IV3c	V3c
18	158	I3b	II3b	III3b	IV3b	V3b
19	126	I3a	II3a	III3a	IV3a	V3a
20	100	I2e	II2e	III2e	IV2e	V2e
21	79	I2d	II2d	III2d	IV2d	V2d
22	63	I2c	II2c	III2c	IV2c	V2c
23	50	I2b	II2b	III2b	IV2b	V2b
24	40	I2a	II2a	III2a	IV2a	V2a
25	32	I1e	III1e	III1e	IV1e	V1e
26	25	I1d	III1d	III1d	IV1d	V1d
27	20	I1c	III1c	III1c	IV1c	V1c
28	16	I1b	III1b	III1b	IV1b	V1b
29	13	I1a	III1a	III1a	IV1a	V1a
30	10		I1e	I2e	III1e	IV1e
31	8		I1d	I2d	III1d	IV1d
32	6		I1c	I2c	III1c	IV1c
33	5		I1b	I2b	III1b	IV1b
34	4		I1a	I2a	III1a	IV1a
35	3.2			I1e	I2e	III1e
36	2.5			I1d	I2d	III1d
37	2.0			I1c	I2c	III1c
38	1.6			I1b	I2b	III1b
39	1.3			I1a	I2a	III1a
40	1.0				I1e	I2e
41	0.8				I1d	I2d
42	0.6				I1c	I2c
43	0.5				I1b	I2b
44	0.4				I1a	I2a
45	0.32					I1e
46	0.25					I1d
47	0.20					I1c
48	0.16					I1b
49	0.13					I1a
50	0.10					I4e
51	0.08					I4d

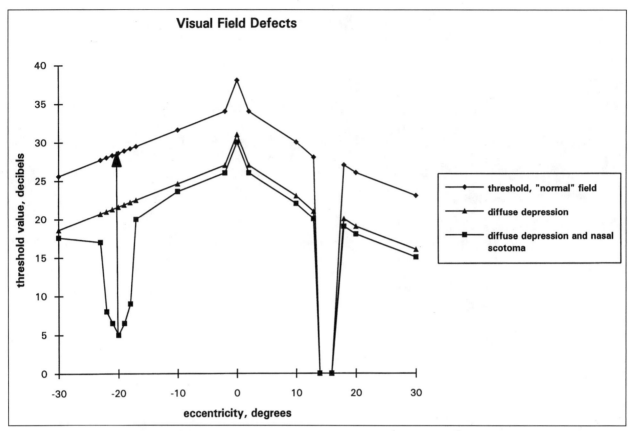

Figure 1-8. Defects in the visual field.

Concepts of Normal in Visual Field Testing

For most clinical applications, "normal" refers to the absence of disease. The concept of normality may be different when dealing with measurable parameters. Values than can be measured in a population can be designated as abnormal when they differ from the average value by some arbitrary amount. For most measurements, the range of normal encompasses 95% of the values falling within two standard deviations on either side of the mean (assuming a statistically normal or "bell-shaped" distribution). Other criteria can be applied for parameters whose measurements are not normally distributed. The key point is that measurements of certain individual's parameters, be it height, weight, blood pressure, intraocular pressure, or the shape and height of the island of vision, may be designated as statistically abnormal (ie, the measurement falls more than two standard deviations from the population mean for that parameter, yet no disease is present). As will be repeated many times, the interpretation of any measurement must be made in the clinical context, taking into consideration all aspects of the patient before deciding on a diagnosis or instituting a change in therapy.

With respect to visual field testing, normal refers to an absence of deviations from expected height and shape of the island of vision. When looking at an isopter plot of a Goldmann field, for example (see bottom of Figure 1-2), it is expected to see a series of concentric ovals drawn around fixation with their greatest extent on the temporal side and decreasing in diameter as the stimulus size becomes smaller and/or dimmer. This "expected" plot is our concept of normal, and a decrease in the size of the ovals, a change in their shape, or the appearance of black spots inside the ovals would lead to the conclusion that the visual field was abnormal. Indeed, there exist "normal" isopter plots, adjusted for age, that can be overlaid onto a patient's visual field plot for comparison of the size and shape of the isopters.

Threshold perimetry generates numerical data, which can be used to produce statistical models of the island of vision. Visual field testing of numerous patients with no ocular disease has given rise to models for the height and shape of the normal island of vision. Statistical analysis of visual fields will be discussed in detail in Chapter 5. The Humphrey Field Analyzer utilizes either the shape model or the height model for displaying abnormalities in the visual field, depending on which software is installed in the machine and which printout options are selected. The optional statistical analysis package, STATPAC, which is discussed in detail in Chapter 5, uses normal threshold values for comparison to a patient's measurements, thus comparing the height of the island of vision at each point in the patient's field to the normals. If STATPAC is not used for analyzing the field data, the machine uses the shape model for determining abnormalities. This involves construction of anticipated normal values based on a few initial threshold measurements. The expected normal values are calculated from the shape model, which gives the slope of the island of vision within the region being tested. For example, if a point measures 25 dB, the next peripheral point should show an expected threshold approximately 0.3 dB less for each degree of eccentricity. For a 6° spacing, the next point should be about 23 dB (25 -[0.3 x 6])—if the patient measures 15 dB, it would be considered below expected normal by eight decibels. The defect depth printout, discussed later, utilizes this expected island of vision model to display how "abnormal" a particular point is. It may not be easy to determine diffuse depression, however, since the model utilizes shape data and not height data.

Types of Visual Field Tests and Printouts

SCREENING VERSUS THRESHOLD TESTING

Information obtainable on a visual field test is limited by the hardware, operating software, analytical software, and most importantly, the patient's ability to undergo the testing. Perimetry is a difficult task for the majority of healthy people; it may be impossible for some people with illness or physical limitations. Accurate performance during a visual field test requires concentration on a fixation target, perception of a light in the peripheral vision, registration that the light was seen, and initiation of a motor response, culminating in a push of the response button. The pathway from the front of the eye to the tip of the thumb is a long, convoluted neuro-anatomic pathway, subject to interruption and short-circuiting anywhere along the way. Thus, in order to obtain meaningful data, it is necessary to strike a balance between the information desired and the patient's ability to perform adequately on the test in order to obtain that information.

Screening the Visual Field

Basically, two types of examinations are available on the Humphrey Field Analyzer. All tests are described in more detail in Chapter 2. *Screening tests* can be used for a quick assessment as to the presence or absence of visual field abnormalities. The screening tests on the Humphrey Field Analyzer use the individualized island of vision based on the shape model, constructed after determination of a few threshold values. Armed with the expected values, each test point is tested with a stimulus six decibels brighter than expected. If sensitivity is normal at that test point, the patient should respond. Lack of response is considered abnormal sensitivity for that point. Different strategies, described in Chapter 2, are available to characterize the nature of the abnormalities. Screening tests are designed to quickly tell whether or not a field is normal without actually drawing the map. Numerical data is not obtained, and there is no estimation of fluctuation. Also, since the individualized island of vision model is used to generate expected normals, small defects will be missed in a field whose thresholds all lie above the age-corrected normals. Suppose a patient has a five-decibel defect at a few field points, yet his entire hill of vision is otherwise five decibels above the level expected for his age. A screening test comparing only the shape of his island of vision using stimuli six decibels above expected (for shape) would miss the five-decibel focal loss. A patient with an abnormal screening test requires further testing to delineate the nature of the abnormalities. Figure 1-9 is a schematic of suprathreshold screening. For this figure, the lower numbers on the vertical axis represent brighter stimuli (lower decibel numbers = less attenuation of the maximum stimulus). Each point is tested with a stimulus six decibels brighter than expected normal as depicted on the middle curve. At any point in the field where the six-decibel line lies below the patient's island of vision profile, the stimulus will be bright enough to elicit a

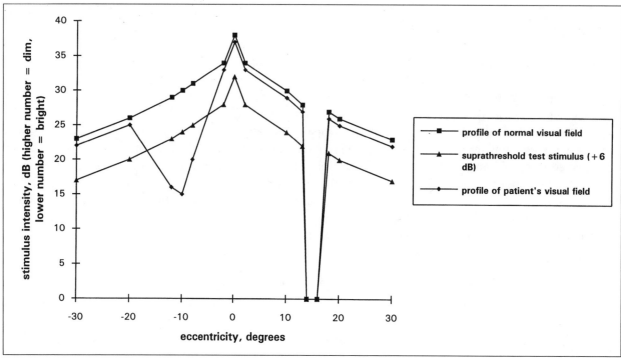

Figure 1-9. Screening tests.

response; if the test stimulus is above the island of vision profile, it will be too dim to elicit a response. Thus, no responses will be obtained in the area of the scotoma centered around -10°. This portion of the field will be labeled as abnormal, but the actual shape of the island in this region has not been determined.

Measuring the Visual Field

Threshold tests actually measure sensitivity at each test point and construct the map of the island of vision. Fluctuation measurements can be made and the numerical data generated can be stored and recalled for analysis with regard to change over time. Population-based normal values can be used for analytical purposes. A threshold test, therefore, would not only detect the overall elevation of the island of vision in the patient example but would detect the isolated five-decibel depressions as well, assuming that the analysis included correction for the diffuse effects. It is recommended that threshold tests be used whenever possible in order to maximize the information obtainable and minimize the need for retesting. Figure 1-10 illustrates how threshold testing can define the contour of the patient's island of vision.

MACHINE OUTPUT: PRINTOUTS

Once a test is completed, the results need to be communicated to the person who ordered the test for use in diagnosis or monitoring ongoing therapy. A variety of options are available on the Humphrey Field Analyzer. Printer options are discussed in Chapter 2, interpretation of visual fields is discussed in detail in Chapter 5.

Screening tests only have one printout option and require no special software. STATPAC does not affect the appearance of the printout from a screening test. What appears on the printout depends on the type of screening test performed and the strategy used. This will be discussed in Chapter 2. Figure 1-11 is an example of a right homonymous hemianopsia in a patient with a left-sided parietal lobe lesion. The results from both eyes are shown. The test was performed with the "quantify defects" strategy. The numbers represent defect depth from expected normal based on the shape model of the island of vision.

Assuming that threshold testing has been done, the most important information is the actual threshold measurements. These are displayed in a value table, as shown in Figure 1-12. The value table represents the "truth," that is, it is a display of what the patient actually did. Any other type of printout is some abstraction

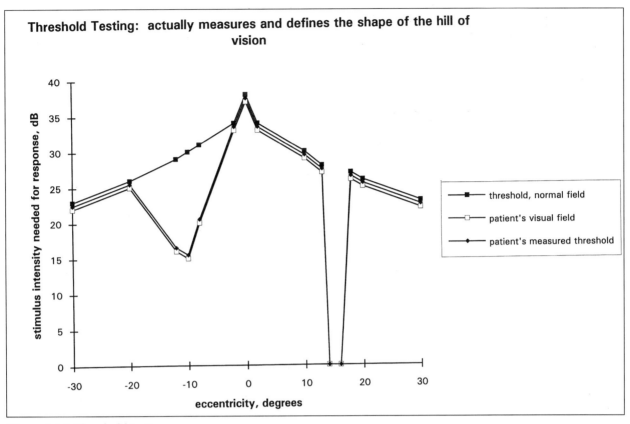

Figure 1-10. Threshold tests.

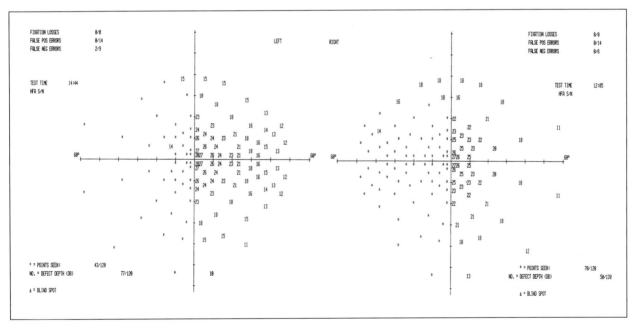

Figure 1-11. Sample printout from a screening test.

Figure 1-12. The value table printout.

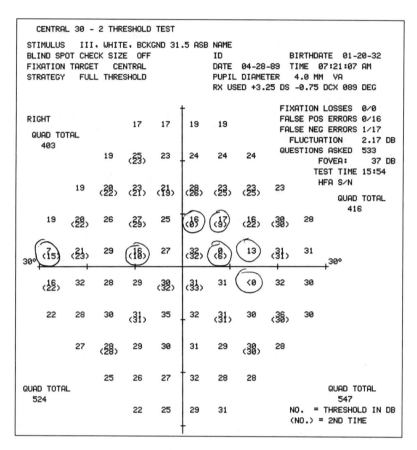

of the truth, requiring manipulation of the data in some manner. Each number on the value table is an actual threshold determination; any points that have had threshold determined more than once will have the repeat measurements indicated in brackets below the first measurement. The interpretation of a value table printout involves scanning the numbers for low values (eg, less than 10 dB) and comparing points to neighboring points, looking for larger differences than would be expected. Such points are circled in Figure 1-12, and the pattern of the depressed points is suggestive of a superior arcuate scotoma.

To demonstrate how the island of vision is affected by areas of decreased sensitivity, the threshold values in Figure 1-12 have been plotted against their (X, Y) coordinates. A topographical map of this plot is shown in Figure 1-13. This type of printout is not available on the Humphrey Field Analyzer, but software packages are available from other sources that are capable of generating these three-dimensional maps. These will be discussed in Chapter 9. In this figure, the island has been rotated and tilted down slightly to allow a view directly into the "canyon," resulting from the depressed sensitivity in the superior arcuate area. The arrow points to the area of depression from the surface.

Another way to display visual field information is by showing the depth of any identified defects. Using the individualized island of vision, or shape model, the algebraic difference between measured value and expected value is calculated and displayed on a grid corresponding to the location of the test points. An example is given in Figure 1-14. This is the same patient as in Figure 1-12. Any point falling within four decibels of expected has the small open circle displayed; points deviating by more than four decibels will have the difference printed. The larger the defect depth, the more severe the abnormality. Remember that this printout is showing depth from expected values, not age-corrected normals.

A graphical or symbolic representation of the threshold data can be given in the form of a "graytone" printout. The arcuate defect present in the patient shown in Figure 1-12 is accentuated by the graytone printout shown in Figure 1-15 and corresponds to the canyon in Figure 1-13. Each number in the value table can be assigned a symbol and the symbol substituted for the number on the printout. The symbols cover a range of decibel values; the translation information for threshold values to graytone symbols is always printed at the bottom of every printout from the Humphrey Field Analyzer. The lower the sensitivity of a field point,

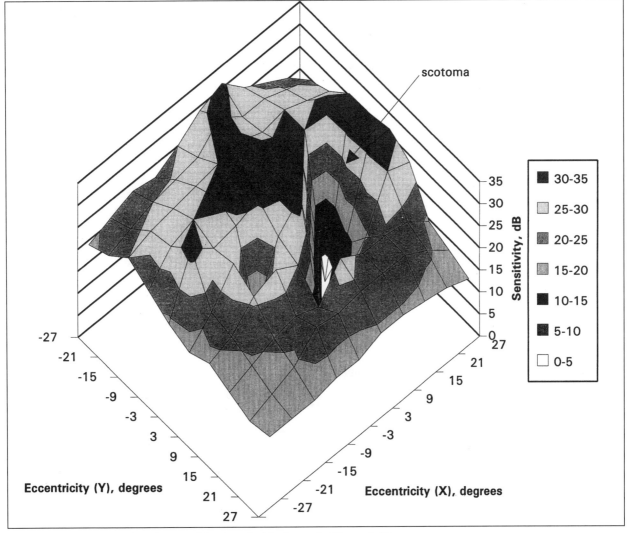

Figure 1-13. A topographical map of the thresholds shown in Figure 1-12.

the darker the symbol used to represent it, so that areas of decreased sensitivity appear dark on the printout and those with good sensitivity will appear lighter. Graytone printouts must be interpreted with caution. They appear to represent the entire field, but only a limited number of points have actually been tested. Areas in between test points have been filled in by interpolation. The graytone may also falsely lead one to suspect a significant defect is present when there really isn't one. This "artifact of graytone construction" is discussed in Chapter 5. The graytone may be used to hone in on areas of the field showing defects or to show the patient where problems are, but it should not be relied on by itself for interpretation. Value table measurements and departures from normal are more useful for accurate interpretation.

For convenience, the Humphrey Field Analyzer provides a printout containing all three printouts on one page, as shown in Figure 1-16. The "three-in-one" printout contains the graytone at the top, the defect depth printout in the lower left, and the value table in the lower right. Having all the information present in one place is useful for purposes of interpretation.

If desired, profile cuts through the island of vision may be printed. Figure 1-17 is a cut through the 30-210 (-30)° meridian. This meridian was chosen to include the superior nerve fiber bundle defect. It appears as a large depression below the surface of the island of vision at 10°. This type of printout is not as clinically useful as the others, but it is available.

If the optional STATPAC analytical software is installed, the printout of a single field will appear as illustrated in Figure 1-18. Extensive discussion of STATPAC is given in Chapter 5.

Figure 1-14. The defect depth printout.

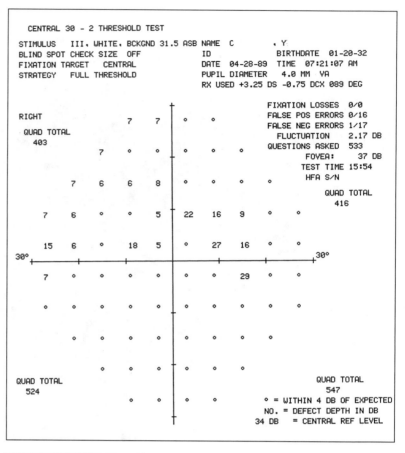

Figure 1-15. The graytone printout.

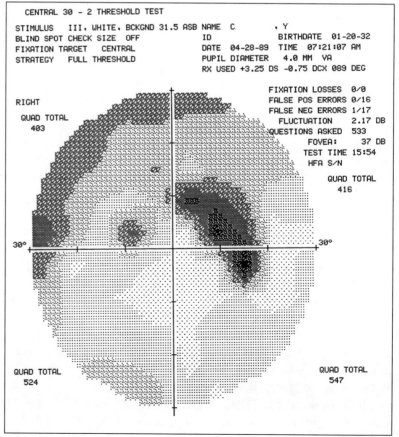

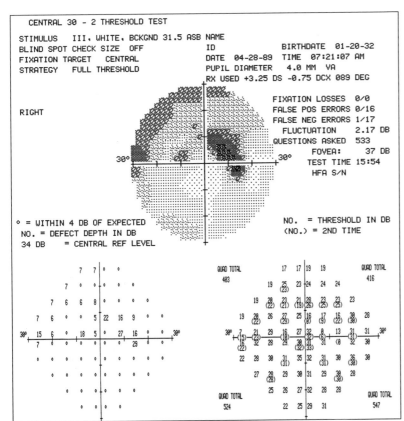

Figure 1-16. The three-in-one printout.

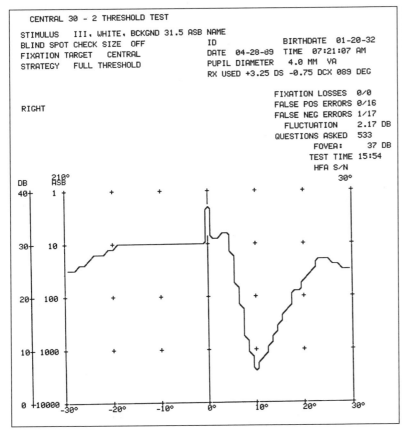

Figure 1-17. A profile cut through the 30° to 210° meridian of the visual field shown in Figure 1-12.

Figure 1-18. The STATPAC printout.

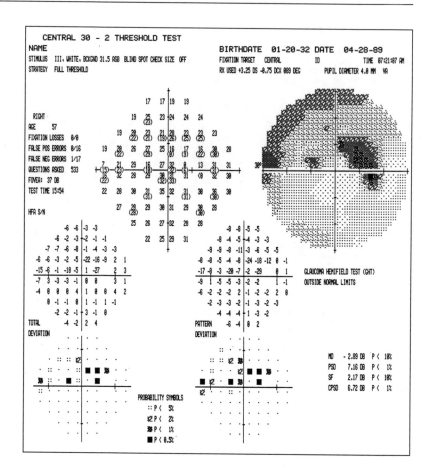

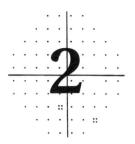

The Humphrey Field Analyzer

Introduction

An understanding of all the capabilities of the Humphrey Field Analyzer is essential for using the machine and acquiring appropriate and meaningful visual field information. Knowledge of the test selection options allows the practitioner to make the correct choices needed to obtain the desired information about a patient. Knowledge of how the machine works and how the various tests are performed allows the perimetrist to troubleshoot the instrument when necessary and help the patient perform a test in a manner that maximizes the chance of providing the clinician with useful information. This chapter discusses the actual "nuts and bolts" of the Humphrey Field Analyzer.

There are two series of Humphrey Field Analyzers. The original series includes models in the 600 series. The Humphrey Field Analyzer (HFA) II series includes models 730, 740, 745, and 750.

Humphrey Field Analyzer 600 Series

PHYSICAL DESCRIPTION OF THE MACHINE

The Humphrey Field Analyzer is a static threshold perimeter that uses a computer-controlled projection system. Contained within the instrument are an illuminated projection bowl, a projector system, a computer to control all aspects of the testing, magnetic media storage devices, and a cathode ray tube (CRT), which allows the perimetrist to interact with the machine.

Measuring 39 inches wide, 19 inches deep, and 34 inches high, it can be set up in a space as small as four by five feet, allowing room for the patient and technician. The machine is placed on a table containing a motorized height adjustment mechanism. The physical location of the instrument as part of the overall perimetry system is discussed in Chapter 3. Figure 2-1 is a schematic of the overall machine design. The top of the figure is the front view, and the bottom is the back view. Refer to this figure in order to locate the various components described below. Note that there may be some variation between the figure and the appearance of your machine, depending on the model. When in doubt, refer to your user's manual.

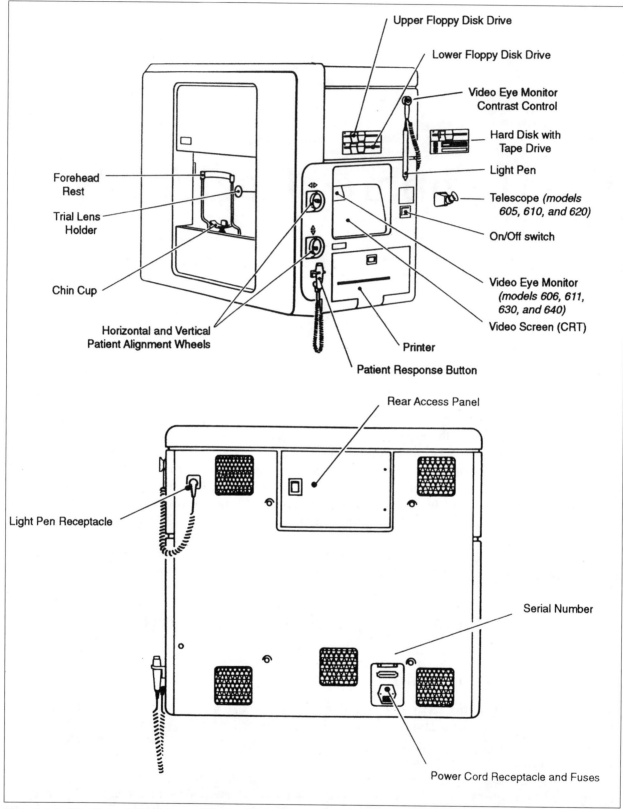

Figure 2-1. Diagram of the front and back of the Humphrey Field Analyzer (adapted with permission from *Field Analyzer Owner's Manual*; San Leandro, Calif: Humphrey Instruments, Inc; 1991).

Visual Field Testing Parameters

The Humphrey Field Analyzer was designed to conform to the standards of the Goldmann perimeter. The projection bowl is 33 cm in radius, which is important for picking the appropriate optical correction for performing a test. The background illumination is 31.5 asb (apostilbs), and is provided by light bulbs that are located at the front of the projection bowl at the 3 and 9 o'clock positions. The bulb housings are covered with diffusing filters. Located in the far upper left-hand side of the bowl is a light meter, which is used at the time of machine start-up to calibrate the intensities of the background and available stimuli. In the center of the bowl is a small fixation light. Models equipped with a video eye monitor have a small television camera built into the fixation point that projects an image of the patient's eye onto the CRT. Just below the fixation light are two sets of four small lamps arranged in concentric diamonds that are used as fixation targets during determination of foveal threshold and as paracentral fixation targets for patients who have lost central vision.

Test stimuli are projected into the bowl by a projector located just above the bowl opening. The projector is moved by a pair of stepper motors under the control of the computer. One motor controls movement in the horizontal direction and the other in the vertical. Later models of the machine utilize a "quiet board," which moves the projector in smaller increments compared to the control board found in the older machines, resulting in less internal noise. Theoretically, less projector noise will result in fewer false positives, as discussed in Chapter 5.

As in the Goldmann perimeter, a shutter is opened to project the stimulus. The default stimulus is a Goldmann size III (four square millimeters), although stimulus sizes I (.25 square millimeters), II (one square millimeters), IV (16 square millimeters), and V (64 square millimeters) are also available. In addition to the standard white stimulus, red, blue, and green stimuli can be selected. The stimulus intensity can be varied from 0.008 to 10,000 asb (63 to 0 dB), representing a range of more than six log units. The range is somewhat lower when color stimuli are used. Stimulus size and color defaults can be changed and stored on the user-defined menu, as discussed later in this chapter.

Displays and Controls

The Humphrey perimeter displays information on a green CRT, located on the left side of the instrument when viewed from the back. Touching "hot spots" on the screen with a light pen enters commands and data. Following the initialization process after powering up the instrument, the main menu will be displayed on the screen, as shown in Figure 2-2. From this initial screen, the perimetrist can select tests to be performed, make use of the data stored on disk, enter new patient data, or alter the instrument's configuration (eg, choosing between printers). If the user-defined menu is utilized, it will be the initial screen seen upon power-up.

In the center of the bowl opening are the patient's chin rest and forehead rest. The height of the table is adjusted to allow the patient's forehead to comfortably contact the rest. The patient's position can be adjusted using the horizontal and vertical alignment wheels on the side of the machine to the left of the video screen. Proper alignment is obtained when the patient's pupil is centered in the telescope mires (models 605, 610, and 620) or between the hash marks in the video eye monitor on the CRT, if so equipped. The patient responds to projected stimuli by means of a hand-held response button that connects to the machine just below the patient alignment wheels.

A lens holder is provided for placement of correcting lenses used to focus the eye onto the interior of the bowl. The lens holder is attached to the right-hand side of the bowl opening. There is an adjustment knob for positioning the lens close to the patient's eye. Positioning of the patient and correcting lens is discussed in detail in Chapter 4.

Computer and Data Storage

The Humphrey perimeter uses an internal computer for all aspects of data entry, patient testing, and printing results. There is no need for an external personal computer unless using optional software for the display of patient results.

Figure 2-2. Humphrey Field Analyzer main menu.

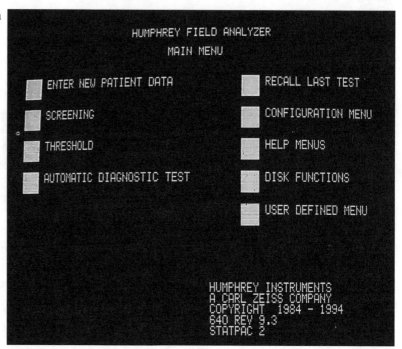

Test results and patient identification data are stored on magnetic media. There are two data storage options: dual floppy disks or single floppy and a hard disk with a streamer tape back-up. Floppy disks can store between 130 and 180 tests. The hard disk can store about 33,000 tests. Formatting floppy disks and the hard drive are proprietary to Humphrey such that data disks cannot be read by any other computer without additional software. The tape back-up is used to restore data to the hard disk in the event of hard disk failure. Frequent back-ups and multiple copies of patient data are highly recommended to prevent data loss.

Output

Printing functions are carried out from the CRT using the light pen. Visual field results, disk directories, and, with later versions of the operating software, patient reminders regarding the need for follow-up examinations can all be generated. Printing results can be done at the conclusion of the examination or at the operator's convenience. Software options allow for printing multiple tests from the disk so that, if desired, an entire day's worth of printing (or more, up to 250 examinations) can be done by selecting the desired tests from the disk and printing with one command.

The Humphrey perimeter contains an internal dot matrix printer. The paper opening is just below the CRT. Printing is on a continuous roll of paper, which allows for multiple tests to be printed on a single long sheet (with the appropriate print option). The paper may be divided into appropriate length sheets by tearing across the upper edge of the opening as it emerges from the printer.

An RS232C serial port is located just above the power cord on the back of the unit. This port can be used to connect an optional laser printer. Redirecting the output to the laser printer is accomplished by changing the set-up parameters using the light pen. The internal printer remains available, thus printing can be accomplished with either printer. There are a few differences in the appearance of the output, especially for the overview analysis and glaucoma change analysis printouts. The laser printer can only fit three fields on an 8½ x 11-inch page. Unless otherwise noted, all of the examples in this book were printed using a peripheral laser printer.

The serial port can also be use to exchange visual field data between Humphrey Field Analyzers or to send data to an external computer. Configuring data transmission is accomplished through the CRT and the light pen. Additional software is required to make use of the field data on other computers. Humphrey, as well as several other vendors, have software programs that are designed to display, print, and assist the practitioner in interpretation of visual field data from the perimeter on a personal computer. Several of these programs will be discussed in Chapter 9.

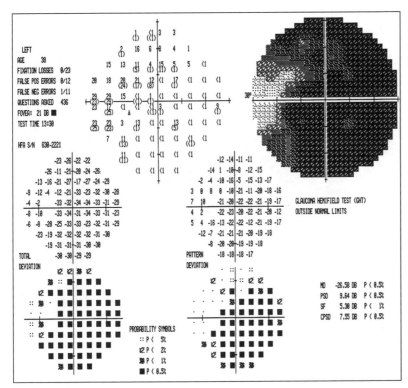

Figure 2-3. Threshold field in a patient with severe visual field loss. Note areas with values recorded as < one, indicating the projector bulb needs to be changed.

MACHINE START-UP PROCEDURES

When the Humphrey perimeter is turned on at the beginning of the day, a series of internal checks begin. The computer memory and software are tested to be sure they are intact. The CRT will display a message that a "RAM" test is being performed. The background illumination in the bowl is measured by the internal light meter and the projector is tested, both for accuracy of projection and for brightness of the maximum stimulus. A message will be displayed on the CRT if a bulb needs to be replaced. Other fault conditions will result in a message display and instructions.

When the projector bulb is no longer able to project a 10,000 asb stimulus, it will still allow testing to continue. This condition can be identified from a threshold test where the patient did not respond to the brightest stimulus available. Under normal circumstances, a point at which no response was obtained is indicated on the printout by a threshold value of < 0. When the projector bulb is no longer able to generate a 10,000 asb stimulus (0 dB attenuation), the printout will show the value in decibels of the maximum stimulus that it was able to project, as is illustrated in Figure 2-3. Since the machine could not generate 10,000 asb, the maximum available due to impending bulb failure is indicated on the printout (in this case one decibel, or 7493 asb), and the fact that the patient didn't respond to that stimulus is indicated by the "<" sign. Should values other than < 0 appear on the printouts, the projector bulb should be changed as soon as possible.

If using the optional laser printer, the printer must be initialized in addition to the perimeter. This is accomplished during the printer set-up. Another brief initialization takes place before the first printout of the day. It is important to turn the printer off before the perimeter at the end of the day and turn it on before the perimeter at the start of the day in order to avoid losing the initialization information. Taping a reminder of the power-up and down sequence to the machine can avoid the need to go through the lengthy printer set-up process.

MAINTENANCE

The Humphrey Field Analyzer has proven to be very reliable and the need for repairs minimal. Down time has fortunately been almost nonexistent. Maintenance requirements are also minimal, and it is recommended that the user's manual be followed. Remember when changing the projector bulb to never contact

Figure 2-4. Location of the EPROMs containing the software.

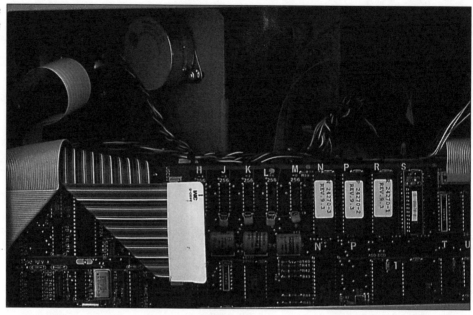

the bulb itself, as this may affect the life of the bulb and its obtainable brightness. Remember also to periodically check the focus of the stimulus as outlined in the manual.

Above all else, routinely back up patient data. If using the hard drive system, keep duplicate copies on floppy disks and back-up with the streamer tape weekly. If using the floppy drive system, make sure that two copies of every test are made. Further recommendations for data storage are given in Chapter 3.

SOFTWARE

Software is the term used for the internal instruction set that controls the instrument. The software for the Humphrey Field Analyzer includes instructions for the initialization process, various screen menus, test array patterns, testing strategies, test performance, statistical analysis, printing, and data storage. The software is not loaded into the instrument by means of floppy disks, as in a personal computer; instead it is contained in computer memory chips called EPROMs, usually installed at the factory . These chips are replaced when the software is upgraded. Figure 2-4 is a photograph showing the location of the EPROM chips with the door to the back of the instrument open (older models of the Humphrey perimeter have a different back panel that must to be removed to allow access to the chips).

The sockets housing the program chips are labeled "N," "P," "R," and "S." Newer models of the perimeter use 16-pin sockets, and the chips are capable of storing more information. The newer models will only require the "N," "P," and "R" chips for all of the operating instructions. The "S" socket is reserved for FAST-PAC. Older models may use 14-pin sockets and require all four chips. Memory chips are also used to store configuration information, for example, the user-defined menu.

Several software options are available for the Humphrey perimeter. STATPAC is an optional software package that contains a number of statistical tools to assist the clinician in evaluating visual field test results. STATPAC 2 is the current version of STATPAC and includes additional glaucoma analysis. FASTPAC is another software option designed to decrease test-taking time. FASTPAC will be discussed later in this chapter. STATPAC is discussed in detail in Chapter 5.

A variety of test options are available on the Humphrey Field Analyzer. As discussed in Chapter 1, the two main categories of tests are screening tests and threshold tests. All tests have three things in common: they consist of an array of points, a strategy for testing those points, and a series of catch trials used to assess reliability. Because of the large number of possible combinations of arrays and strategies, a user-defined menu can be created with up to eight tests defined for use. If a user-defined menu has been created, it is the first screen displayed following initialization. Tests not defined on the user-defined menu are still available using the standard menus. Figure 2-5 is an example of a user-defined menu. All parameters of a test can be

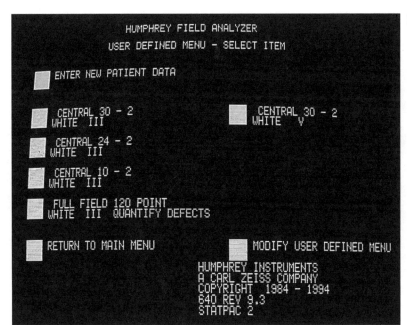

Figure 2-5. User-defined menu.

specified and stored as an item on the user-defined menu. For example, saving nonstandard parameters with an array and test strategy saves many steps in configuring the machine to perform a test. Having a 10-2 with a red test object already on the menu saves going through the "change parameters" screen when testing a patient with those parameters. A typical user-defined menu will include a central 30° test with full threshold strategy using stimulus size III, another set the same way but with stimulus size V, a 10-2 test, and a screening test. Since it is user defined, it should be set up for the types of situations most commonly encountered in your clinical practice. Test selection and various parameters will be discussed in Chapter 4.

The various test point arrays and strategies for screening and threshold tests are discussed below. Three measures of reliability are performed during all visual field tests. These are estimates of fixation loss, false positive response rate, and false negative response rate. The default is to test fixation losses, however, the user can turn this off. These measures of reliability will be discussed in detail in Chapter 5. Briefly, fixation losses are indicated by a patient response to a stimulus projected into where the machine previously located the blind spot, false positive responses are patient responses to a nonprojected stimulus, and false negative responses are patient failures to respond to the brightest stimulus projected into an area previously determined to have some sensitivity. A running tally of the catch trials is kept in the lower right-hand corner of the CRT as the test is being performed. Each is reported as a fraction, with the denominator representing the total number for that catch trial and the numerator indicating the number of times the patient "fell for it." Each time a false response or fixation loss occurs, the machine will beep and the numerator (as well as the denominator) for that measure will increase by one. The operator should be continuously monitoring these during the test, and re-instruct the patient as necessary. This is discussed in detail in Chapter 4.

Screening Tests

Screening tests are designed to quickly determine whether or not a field is "normal." These tests take less time to perform than the threshold tests, but they provide less information in exchange. When field deficits are located with a screening test, follow-up threshold testing is indicated in most situations to quantify the defect found and to provide a baseline for later statistical comparison. Screening tests are most useful in asymptomatic patients with disease processes in which visual field defects are expected to be found. A screening test can also be useful as a first exam in a patient who is expected to have difficulty performing a threshold test.

Table 2-1

SCREENING FIELD TEST PATTERNS FOR THE HFA 600 SERIES

Test Pattern	Number of Test Points	Typical Test Time (minutes per eye)
Glaucoma Tests		
Armaly central	84	5 to 6
Armaly full field	98	7 to 8
Nasal step	14	2 to 3
Central 30 Tests		
Central 40-point	40	2 to 4
Central 76-point†	76	3 to 5
Central 80-point	80	3 to 5
Central 166-point	166	13 to 14
Peripheral Tests		
Peripheral 68-point‡	68	5 to 6
Full field 81-point	81	6 to 7
Full field 120-point	120	6 to 8
Full field 246-point	246	14 to 15
Custom Tests		
Points can be added to any test pattern above or used alone		

† This test array is the same as the 30-2 threshold pattern

‡ This test array is the same as the 30/60-2 threshold pattern

Screening Test Point Arrays

There are 11 test patterns available on the screening test menu. In addition, there is a custom pattern option. Table 2-1 lists the available screening test arrays that may be available (depending on the version of software) grouped by type of screening pattern. The glaucoma screening patterns emphasize points surrounding the horizontal meridian with the largest concentration of points in the nasal field. Humphrey defines central tests as out to 30° and full field tests as out to 60°, therefore the central 30° screening tests examine a variety of points in the central field. Among the central screening tests, the central 76-point screening test is particularly useful because the points in its array are the same as is tested in the central 30-2 threshold test. Similarly, the points in the nasal step screening test are in the same positions as the nasal step threshold test. None of the other central screening test patterns have corresponding full threshold tests. The peripheral test patterns provide a variety of arrays that examine the visual field beyond the central 30°. The peripheral 68-point test pattern uses the same pattern as in the peripheral 30/60-2 threshold test.

Screening Test Strategies

The Humphrey Field Analyzer has four screening test strategies available: threshold related, three zone, quantify defects, and single intensity. All four strategies are available for each of the screening test arrays. While the instrument defaults to the threshold-related strategy when screening tests are selected from the main menu, an alternative screening strategy can be established as the default in the user-defined menu.

In the threshold-related strategy, the Humphrey perimeter determines the patient's threshold (as discussed in Chapter 1) at four paracentral points (one in each quadrant) during the first part of the test. It uses these values to calculate a "central reference level" and, using the "shape" model of the island of vision described in Chapter 1, expected normal threshold values for each point in the array. In the screening phase of the test, each point in the selected test pattern is exposed to a stimulus six decibels brighter than the expected threshold for that point. Points not seen with the first stimulus are retested with the same stimulus intensity later in the test. Upon completion of the examination, tested points are either labeled with an open circle, indicating the patient responded, or with a black box, indicating the patient failed to respond upon two

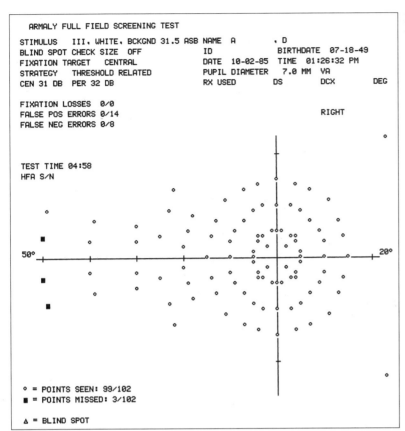

Figure 2-6. Armaly full field screening test using the threshold-related strategy.

presentations of the suprathreshold stimulus. Figure 2-6 is an example of a threshold-related test. A legend is given at the bottom of the printout defining the symbols.

The three-zone strategy begins in the same manner as the threshold-related strategy. The central reference level is determined and defects are located using the same six decibels brighter than expected method. Points that are not seen following the second stimulus are retested with a maximum (10,000 asb) stimulus. Points missed with stimuli six decibels brighter than expected but seen with the maximum stimulus are marked with an "X" and labeled as relative defects. Points missed with the maximum stimulus are marked with the black box and labeled as absolute defects. Note that the test does not really prove that there is total lack of sensitivity, only that the points so labeled were not seen with a stimulus intensity of 10,000 asb. Figure 2-7 is an example of a three-zone test.

Like the three-zone test, the quantify defects screening test begins by determining the central reference level. Points in the array are tested with a stimulus six decibels brighter than the patient's expected visual field profile based upon the test initialization process. Points not seen on the second projection of the six decibels brighter than expected stimulus have threshold determined as described in Chapter 1. When the test results are printed, points seen with the stimulus six decibels brighter than expected are labeled as seen, again with an open circle. Points that required threshold determinations are labeled with the defect depth. The defect depth is the difference between the expected threshold value based on the constructed patient profile and the measured threshold value. Figure 2-8 is an example of a screening test using the quantify defects strategy.

The single-intensity test is the fastest test strategy available. Each point in the selected grid is tested with the specified stimulus intensity, regardless of its location in the field. Missed points are tested a second time at the same stimulus intensity. Points are labeled as seen or missed, as demonstrated in Figure 2-9. If desired, the stimulus intensity can be set to a different value using the test configuration menu; the default value is 24 dB. Some states require specified Goldmann isopter mapping as part of disability ratings. If an isopter is specified, it can be converted to a decibel value using Table 1-1 and the single intensity screening test performed with that specific value.

Figure 2-7. Full field 120-point screening test using the three-zone strategy. Points labeled with an "X" were missed with a suprathreshold stimulus but seen with the maximum (10,000 asb) stimulus.

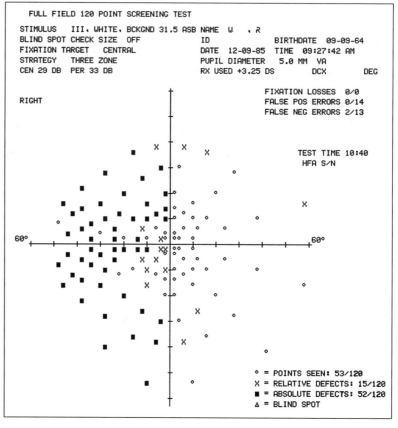

Figure 2-8. Full field 120-point screening test using the quantify defects strategy. Compare this to the three-zone strategy test in the same patient in Figure 2-7. Points missed with a suprathreshold stimulus have their threshold determined. The values displayed are the calculated defect depth.

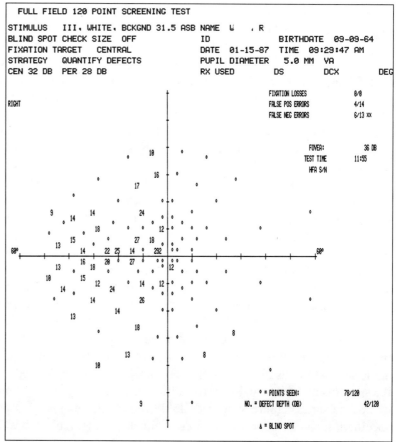

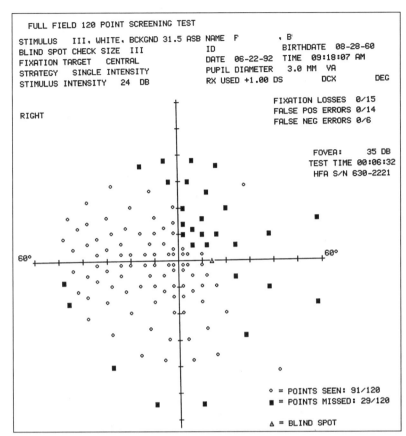

FULL FIELD 120 POINT SCREENING TEST

STIMULUS   III, WHITE, BCKGND 31.5 ASB   NAME P   , B
BLIND SPOT CHECK SIZE III   ID   BIRTHDATE 08-28-60
FIXATION TARGET   CENTRAL   DATE 06-22-92 TIME 09:18:07 AM
STRATEGY   SINGLE INTENSITY   PUPIL DIAMETER   3.0 MM VA
STIMULUS INTENSITY   24 DB   RX USED +1.00 DS   DCX   DEG

                                                    FIXATION LOSSES 0/15
RIGHT   FALSE POS ERRORS 0/14
                                                     FALSE NEG ERRORS 0/6

                                                     FOVEA: 35 DB
                                                     TEST TIME 00:06:32
                                                     HFA S/N 630-2221

60°   60°

                                                 ○ = POINTS SEEN: 91/120
                                                 ■ = POINTS MISSED: 29/120

                                                 △ = BLIND SPOT

Figure 2-9. Full field 120-point screening test using the single-intensity strategy.

Software versions with FASTPAC include an alternate method for determining the visual field profile to compare the patient with during screening tests. This alternate method uses an age-related field profile instead of determining the expected normal profile from the initialization process. Eliminating the four threshold determinations at the beginning of the test reduces test-taking time by about one minute on all screening tests. The age reference strategy can be selected from the options listed in the "change parameters" menu if it is available. Once selected, the option remains in effect for all screening tests performed until it is deselected or the instrument is turned off. The age-related reference levels do not apply to the single intensity screen.

Threshold Tests

Threshold tests actually measure threshold at each test point using the methods described in Chapter 1 and provide quantitative information about a patient's visual field. The data obtained from one examination can be compared with previous and subsequent exams. Statistical analysis of the visual field data is available to assist the clinician in diagnostic and therapeutic decision making. These tests generally take longer to perform than the screening tests, and some patients may find them too difficult to perform without adequate supervision from the technician. Even when a threshold test is the most appropriate exam, a screening field may be useful as a tool to teach the patient how to perform a test on the Humphrey perimeter.

A variety of options exist for displaying the results of threshold tests. These are discussed in Chapter 5. The raw data obtained in the threshold tests consist of threshold values for each point tested in the array as well as measures of reliability and short-term fluctuation. Foveal threshold can be determined as well. The various display options present the data in different manners and reduce portions of it into statistical indices to facilitate interpretation.

In the threshold tests, there is an option to determine threshold at the point of fixation. The value obtained from this measurement is called the foveal threshold. Measurement of foveal threshold is selected from the "change parameters" screen. The CRT flashes a message reminding the perimetrist to direct the patient to

Table 2-2

THRESHOLD FIELD TEST PATTERNS FOR THE HFA 600 SERIES

Test Pattern	Point Density (°)	# Test Points	Typical Test Time (minutes per eye)	Notes
Central Tests				
Central 24-1	6	56	10 to 12	Test points begin on horizontal and vertical meridians
Central 24-2	6	54	10 to 12	Test points straddle the horizontal and vertical meridians
Central 30-1	6	71	12 to 15	Test points begin on horizontal and vertical meridians
Central 30-2	6	76	12 to 15	Test points straddle the horizontal and vertical meridians
Peripheral Tests				
Peripheral 30/60-1	12	63	12 to 15	Test points begin on horizontal and vertical meridians
Peripheral 30/60-2	12	68	12 to 15	Test points straddle the horizontal and vertical meridians
Nasal step	†	14	2 to 3	
Temporal crescent	8.5	37	3 to 4	
Specialty Tests				
Neurological 20	†	16[1]	5 to 6	Test points aligned on either side of the vertical meridian
Neurological 50	†	22[1]	8 to 9	Test points aligned on either side of the vertical meridian
Central 10-2	2	68	10 to 12	Region tested about the same as Amsler grid
Macula	2	16[2]	8 to 10	
Custom Tests				
Points can be added to any of the test patterns above or used alone				

† Test point density decreases with increasing eccentricity
1 Each point has the threshold determined twice
2 Each point has the threshold determined three times

look into the center of the diamond fixation target. A standard threshold determination, as described in Chapter 1, is made at this point by projecting the stimuli into the center of the diamond. Abnormal in some macular and optic nerve disease, *foveal threshold* is also a useful parameter in evaluating the accuracy of the field (patients with normal visual acuity usually have a normal foveal threshold). Abnormalities should prompt the clinician to be certain the test was performed properly, with particular attention paid to the correcting lens. Table 2-2 lists the 12 test patterns available on the threshold test menu.

Test Point Arrays

As with the screening tests, custom patterns can be created as well. The optional statistical packages STATPAC and STATPAC 2 can be used on all the central fields. Discussed in Chapter 5, they provide the clinician with software tools to compare a patient with age-related normal values and to help evaluate changes in the visual fields over time.

The central 24-1 and 24-2, the central 30-1 and 30-2, and the peripheral 30/60-1 and 30/60-2 fields have complementary arrays and can be merged, increasing the point density of these tests. Figure 2-10 illustrates the differences between the 30-1 and 30-2 exams. Note that the 30-1 test points lie along the vertical and horizontal meridians, while the 30-2 test points straddle these meridians. The points in the 24-2 and 30-2 tests are offset from the axes by 3°. The spacing of points from each other in both grids is 6°. Since the diagnosis

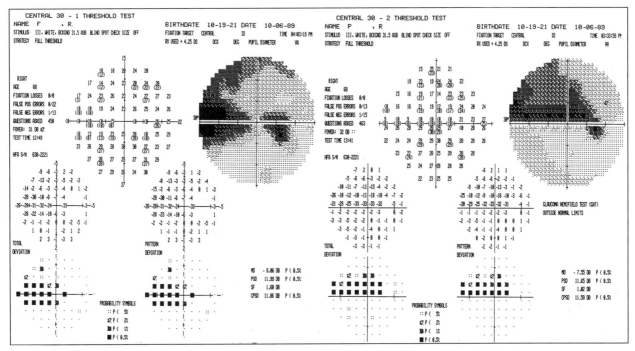

Figure 2-10. Central 30-1 and 30-2 fields. Note the complementary test points.

of glaucoma and neurological diseases frequently relies on finding field defects that do not cross over one or the other of these meridians, the 24-2 and 30-2 tests are more frequently used. The portion of the field tested with the central 10-2 pattern is approximately the same as is evaluated with the Amsler grid.

One printout option for patients who have been tested with both 30-1 and 30-2 tests is to merge the tests together into one printout, as shown in Figure 2-11. The resultant printout has a resolution of 3° since the points of the -1 and -2 points interdigitate. The example is the merger of the examinations shown in Figure 2-10. A peripheral threshold test can also be merged with a central test to give threshold results out to 60°.

Threshold Testing Strategies

Three test strategies are available for determining threshold with the Humphrey Field Analyzer: full threshold, full threshold from prior data, and fast threshold. The latter two methods require previous visual field data and are therefore only available in patients whose fields are being tested over time. A fourth strategy comes with the optional software package FASTPAC.

After mapping the blind spot and determining foveal threshold (if selected), the full-threshold strategy determines threshold at four primary paracentral points. From these values, it constructs an expected field profile for the patient. Threshold determination at each point in the test pattern begins with a stimulus six decibels brighter than is expected to be seen based on the constructed profile. As discussed in Chapter 1, the brightness of subsequent stimuli is changed in accordance with the patient's responses until threshold has been crossed twice. Presentations are made randomly within the test array to decrease the probability of "anticipation" responses. The threshold value assigned is the value midway between the last two stimulus intensities, where threshold was crossed the second time. The machine may determine threshold a second or even third time in a portion of the field where points were found to have abnormal values. Second and third threshold determinations are indicated in parentheses and lie immediately below the first threshold value on the value table in the printout. Examples of threshold printouts with discussion are given in Chapters 1 and 5. Clinical examples may be found in Chapters 6 through 8.

The full threshold from prior data is performed using a visual field profile for the patient that was measured during a previous threshold test. The threshold is determined (as described in Chapter 1) using a stimulus two decibels brighter than the patient's previously determined threshold for each point in the test array as the starting point. This strategy is most valuable for patients with moderate visual field loss; the threshold

Figure 2-11. Result from merging the fields in Figure 2-10. Note that the merged field has a much higher test point density.

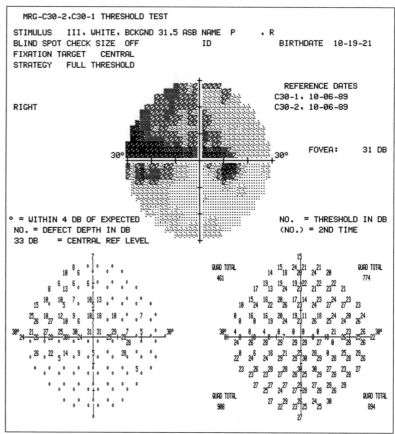

determination requires fewer stimulus presentations, thereby decreasing the test time and reducing patient fatigue. The threshold values determined using this strategy can be used by STATPAC for analysis for changes over time.

The fast-threshold strategy is also performed using previously measured visual field data. A master data file is required. This file is created from one to five full threshold or full threshold from prior data visual fields. Data from this master file are used to determine the stimulus intensity used in the fast-threshold strategy. Each point is tested with a stimulus two decibels brighter than the value in the master file. If seen, the point is assigned the threshold value in the master file. If not seen, the point has threshold determined as described in Chapter 1. While significantly speeding up test time, results from the fast-threshold test cannot be used in STATPAC analysis, nor can they be used in creating a new master file. The problem with the fast strategy is that it will fail to detect an improvement in threshold values since any point that is responded to a two decibels brighter than the assigned value will not have threshold determined. This strategy should be used infrequently and interpreted with caution.

The following steps are used to create a master file:

1. Copy all the fields to be used for the master file to a single disk (floppy or hard).
2. Select "disk functions" from the main menu and then choose "create master file."
3. Choose a disk source that the files are located on.
4. Scroll up or down to locate the desired files and highlight up to five fields.
5. Choose "selection complete." Once the averaging is complete, choose "save on disk." The master file is saved on both floppies or on the floppy and hard disk.

The final threshold strategy, available only as an option, is FASTPAC. FASTPAC reduces the test time for threshold tests by about 40% by measuring threshold with an alternative strategy to the staircase method described in Chapter 1. Instead of changing stimulus intensity by four-decibel steps until the first crossing of threshold and then reversing direction in two-decibel steps, FASTPAC changes the stimulus intensity in three-decibel steps and crosses threshold only once; the threshold value assigned to each tested point in the array lies between the two stimulus intensities where threshold was crossed. The threshold values determined using FASTPAC have been shown to be statistically the same as those found on standard testing. However, because of the wider interval between the stimulus intensities, FASTPAC tends to overestimate short-term fluctuation. Most of the STATPAC data analysis can be performed with tests run using FASTPAC, but the glaucoma change analysis cannot. The standard printouts are available; FASTPAC tests are labeled with the word "FASTPAC" in the upper left corner just below the strategy and patient name. If an instrument has FASTPAC software, it will be found as an option on the "change parameters" menu. Once selected, FAST-PAC is the threshold strategy used until it is deselected or the instrument is turned off and then on again. However, it can be included as a default parameter on a test in the user-defined menu.

Automatic Diagnostic Test

The automatic diagnostic test is available as an intensive screening tool. This test is designed to evaluate the size and depth of defects found during screening. In this test, points missed with a suprathreshold stimulus have threshold determinations made. Up to 10 additional points surrounding each defect are screened using a threshold-related strategy to help determine the size of the defect. If more than 40 points are missed, threshold determinations are not made. Results from this test cannot be used with STATPAC.

Custom Tests

The Humphrey software allows the user to custom design tests. Arrays of points for custom screening can be selected by grids, grids specified by X, Y coordinates, single points, single points by X, Y coordinates, point clusters, and point clusters by X, Y coordinates. Custom threshold tests can also be designed using the same types of point selections, as well as profiles and arcs. Custom tests can be stored and recalled for use from the menus. Custom tests have been used for research purposes, such as exploring the peripheral nasal field for glaucomatous defects not detected in the central 30°, or for "sampling" the visual field as a quick estimate of mean retinal sensitivity. For most clinical situations, the preprogrammed tests are sufficient. In addition, custom points can be added to standard tests following their conclusion in order to further "explore" abnormal areas.

Defaults

With the ability to create a user-defined menu and provide custom point testing, the Humphrey perimeter offers a great deal of flexibility for meeting the needs of the clinician. For reference, the default values for the test parameters are listed in Table 2-3 for the most commonly used screening and threshold tests.

Humphrey Field Analyzer II 700 Series

PHYSICAL DESCRIPTION OF THE MACHINE

Like the original HFA, The Humphrey Field Analyzer II is a static threshold perimeter that uses a computer-controlled projection system. Contained within the instrument are an illuminated projection bowl, a projector system, a computer to control all aspects of the testing, magnetic media storage devices, and a touchscreen grayscale CRT display that allows the perimetrist to interact with the machine. Having a smaller footprint than the original HFA, the HFA II measures 22 3/4 inches wide, 19 inches deep, and 23 5/8 inches high; it can be set up in a space as small as four by five feet, allowing room for the patient and technician. The machine is placed on an adjustable table that is designed to extend to the patient instead of requiring the patient to stretch toward the instrument. Figures 2-12 and 2-13 are schematic diagrams of the overall machine design. The top of Figure 2-12 is the side view and the bottom is the back of the instrument. Figure 2-13 is the front view of the instrument and includes the adjustable table with mounted printer. Refer to these figures in order to locate the various components described below. Note that there may be some variation between the figures and the appearance of your machine, depending upon the model. When in doubt, refer to your user's manual.

Table 2-3
Screening Field Test Patterns for the HFA II

Test Pattern	Number of Test Points	Typical Test Time (minutes per eye)
Glaucoma Tests		
Armaly central	84	5 to 6
Armaly full field	98	7 to 8
Nasal step	14	2 to 3
Central 30 Tests		
Central 40-point	40	2 to 4
Central 76-point†	76	3 to 5
Central 80-point	80	3 to 5
Peripheral Tests		
Peripheral 60-point‡	60	5 to 6
Full field 81-point	81	6 to 7
Full field 120-point	120	6 to 8
Full field 135-point	135	7 to 9
Full field 246-point	246	14 to 15
Superior 36-point	36	2 to 4
Superior 64-point	64	5 to 6
Custom Tests		
Points can be added to any test pattern above or used alone		

† This test array is the same as the 30-2 threshold pattern
‡ This test array is the same as the 60-4 threshold pattern

Visual Field Testing Parameters

Like the Humphrey Field Analyzer, the HFA II was designed to conform to the standards of the Goldmann perimeter. The projection bowl has a 30 cm radius, which is important for picking the appropriate optical correction for performing a test. The bowl has an aspheric design intended to reduce accommodative demand when testing the peripheral visual field. The background illumination is 31.5 asb and is provided by fluorescent light bulbs located at the front of the projection bowl at the two and 10 o'clock positions.

There are three fixation targets. The first is a yellow light in the center of the bowl and is used for most testing. Just below the fixation light are two sets of four small lamps arranged in concentric diamonds that are used as fixation targets during determination of foveal threshold and as paracentral fixation targets for patients who have lost central vision. The video eye monitor consists of a small television camera built into the fixation point, which projects an image of the patient's eye onto the CRT display.

Test stimuli are projected in the same manner as the HFA. In addition to the blind spot method of testing for fixation losses, the HFA II incorporates "gaze-tracking." In this method of monitoring fixation, a light is projected onto the cornea and the position of its reflection is determined. When the eye moves, so does the reflection; the quantity and magnitude of movement away from fixation is measured and recorded on the bottom of the printout. As with fixation loss monitoring, the user can elect to turn off gaze tracking, but it does not add to test time since no additional stimulus presentations are required. The gaze tracker will automatically pause a test if the patient closes the eye or moves away from the head rest, so it is recommended that it be used whenever possible.

Displays and Controls

The HFA II displays information on a grayscale CRT touch screen, located on the left side of the instrument when viewed from the back. Optionally, an external computer monitor may be used. Touching "hot

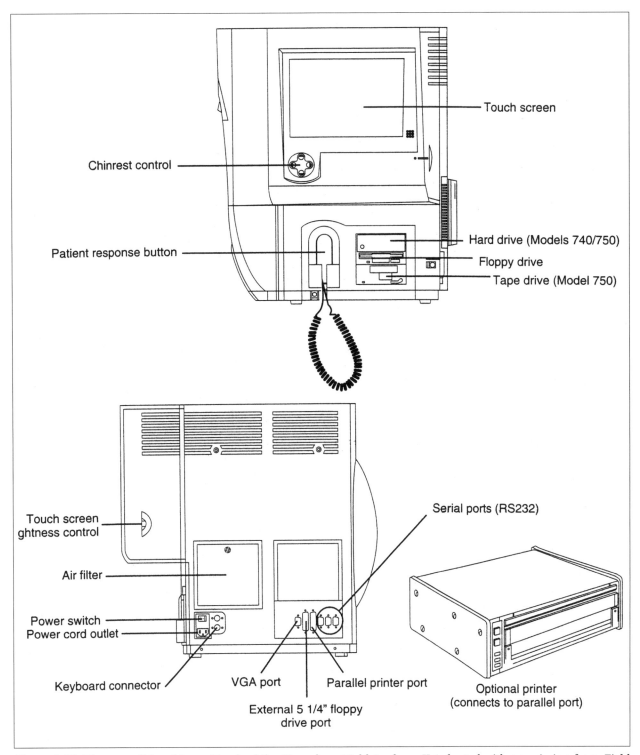

Figure 2-12. Diagram of the side and back of the Humphrey Field Analyzer II (adapted with permission from *Field Analyzer II User's Guide*. Rev A. San Leandro, Calif: Humphrey Instruments, Inc; 1994).

Figure 2-13. Diagram of the front of the Humphrey Field Analyzer II and the table with mounted printer (adapted with permission from *Field Analyzer II User's Guide*. Rev A. San Leandro, Calif: Humphrey Instruments, Inc; 1994).

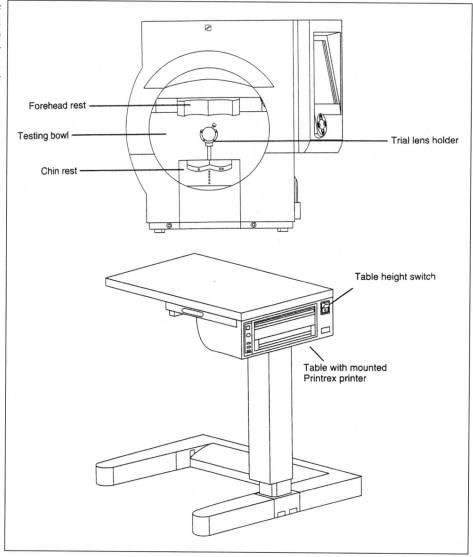

Forehead rest

Testing bowl

Chin rest

Trial lens holder

Table height switch

Table with mounted Printrex printer

spots" on the internal screen with a finger enters commands and data. An external personal computer keyboard may also be used for menu navigation and data entry.

Following the initialization process after powering up the instrument, the main menu will be displayed on the screen, as shown in Figure 2-14. From this initial screen, the perimetrist can select tests to be performed, make use of the data stored on disk, enter new patient data, or alter the instrument's configuration (eg, choosing between printers). If the user-defined menu is utilized, it will be the initial screen seen upon power-up.

In the center of the bowl opening are the patient's chin rest and forehead rest. The chin rest is divided into two cups, one for testing the right eye and one for the left. The height of the table is adjusted to allow the patient's forehead to comfortably contact the headrest. The patient's position can be adjusted using the horizontal and vertical alignment rocker switch on the side of the machine to the left of the video screen. Proper alignment is obtained when the patient's pupil is centered on the target in the video eye monitor in the upper left-hand corner of the CRT screen. The patient responds to projected stimuli by means of a hand-held response button that connects to the machine just below the patient alignment rocker switch. Some models will make automatic adjustments in the position of the chin rest during a test to allow for small head movements.

A lens holder is provided for placement of the lenses used to focus the eye onto the interior of the bowl. The lens holder is attached to the chin rest and can be moved into a storage position when not required. The

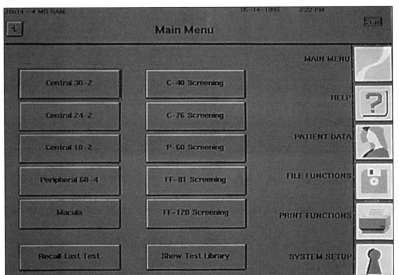

Figure 2-14. Main menu screen of the Humphrey Field Analyzer II. Note the navigation icons on the right-hand side of the touch screen. These are present on every menu on the Humphrey Field Analyzer II and allow the user to return to get online help, enter or modify patient information, use the file functions of the Humphrey Field Analyzer II, print tests, and modify the system set-up, as well as return to the main menu from any screen.

arm of the lens holder can be moved to or away from the patient in order to position the lens close to the patient's eye. Positioning the patient and correcting lens is discussed in detail in Chapter 4.

Computer and Data Storage

The HFA II perimeter uses an internal computer for all aspects of data entry, patient testing, and printing results. There is no need for an external personal computer unless using optional software for the display of patient results.

Test results and patient identification data are stored on magnetic media. All models are equipped with a single 3½-inch floppy drive. The 740 model has a 270 MB (megabyte) hard disk, while the 750 model has a 540 MB hard disk and a streamer tape back-up. Floppy disks can store more than 200 tests, and the hard disk can store more than 200,000 tests. Floppy disks must be initialized prior to use; this can be done by the field analyzer or on any IBM-compatible personal computer that uses 3½-inch high density disks. The tape back-up is used to restore data to the hard disk in the event of hard disk failure. Frequent back-ups and multiple copies of patient data are highly recommended to prevent data loss.

Output

Printing functions are carried out from the CRT touch screen. Visual field results, disk directories, and patient reminders regarding the need for follow-up examinations can all be generated. Printing results can be done at the conclusion of the examination or at the operator's convenience. Software options allow for printing multiple tests from the disk so that, if desired, an entire day's worth of printing can be done by selecting the desired tests from the disk and printing with one command.

The HFA II perimeter stand contains a thermal line printer. The paper opening is just below the tabletop on the technician's side of the stand. Printing is on a continuous roll of paper, which allows for multiple tests to be printed on a single long sheet (with the appropriate print option). The paper may be divided into appropriate length sheets by tearing across the upper edge of the opening as it emerges from the printer.

Ports for connecting various devices to the HFA II are located on same side of the instrument as the power switch and power cord outlet, on the side to the right of the CRT screen. Included are three RS232C serial ports for communication with other instruments. The serial ports are located in the lower right-hand corner. Just to the left of the serial ports is a parallel printer port for attaching a printer. Adjacent to the parallel port is an external 5¼-inch floppy drive port for transferring data to and from field analyzer 600 series models. A VGA port lies to the left of the external floppy drive port and permits the connection of an external monitor. Just to the right of the power switch and power cord outlet lies the keyboard connector port.

Redirecting the output to an external laser printer is accomplished by changing the set-up parameters on the touch screen, disconnecting the printer cable from the thermal printer, and reconnecting it to the external laser printer. The table-mounted thermal line printer cannot be used at the same time as an external laser printer. There are a few differences in the appearance of the output, especially for the overview analysis and glaucoma change analysis printouts. The laser printer can only fit three fields on an 8½ x 11-inch page.

The serial ports can be use to exchange visual field data between Humphrey Field Analyzers or to send data to an external computer. Configuring data transmission is accomplished through touch screens. Additional software is required to make use of the field data on other computers. Humphrey, as well as several other vendors, have software programs that are designed to display, print, and assist the practitioner in interpretation of visual field data from the perimeter on a personal computer. Several of these programs will be discussed in Chapter 9.

MACHINE START-UP PROCEDURES

When the Humphrey perimeter is turned on at the beginning of the day, a series of internal checks begins. The computer memory and software are tested to be sure they are intact. Initially, the instrument will display the model number, software version, and instrument's serial number. The screen will then briefly display the instrument model number again followed by a screen that simply says "startup." During the start-up process, the background illumination in the bowl is measured by the internal light meter, and the projector is tested, both for accuracy of projection and for brightness of the maximum stimulus. A message will be displayed if a bulb needs to be replaced. Other fault conditions will result in a message display and instructions.

When the projector bulb is no longer able to project a maximum stimulus, it will still allow testing to continue. See the discussion earlier in this chapter in the *HFA 600 Series Machine Start-Up Procedures* section for more details.

If using the optional laser printer, the printer must be initialized in addition to the perimeter. This is accomplished during the printer set-up. Another brief initialization takes place before the first printout of the day. It is important to turn the printer off before the perimeter at the end of the day and turn it on before the perimeter at the start of the day in order to avoid losing the initialization information. Taping a reminder of the sequence of power-up and down to the machine can avoid the need to go through the lengthy printer set-up process.

MAINTENANCE

The Humphrey Field Analyzer II has proven to be very reliable, and the need for repairs is minimal. Down time has fortunately been almost nonexistent. Maintenance requirements are also minimal, and it is recommended that the user's manual be followed. Remember when changing the projector bulb to never touch the bulb itself, as this may affect the life of the bulb and its obtainable brightness. Remember also to periodically check the focus of the stimulus, as outlined in the manual.

Above all else, routinely back-up patient data. If using the hard drive system, keep duplicate copies on floppy disks and back-up with the streamer tape weekly. If using the floppy drive system, make sure that two copies of every test are made. Further recommendations for data storage are given in Chapter 3.

Software

The software for the Humphrey Field Analyzer II includes instructions for the initialization process, various screen menus, test array patterns, testing strategies, statistical analysis, printing, and data storage. Unlike the 600 series, upgraded software for the 700 series is loaded into the instrument by means of floppy disks, as with personal computers.

As in the 600 series, a variety of test options are available on the HFA II. The screening and thresholding strategies are, for the most part, the same in the two series. Notable exceptions include short-wavelength automated perimetry (SWAP), available on models 745 and 750, and the Swedish Interactive Thresholding Algorithm (SITA). These two techniques will be discussed in Chapter 9. Most of the test arrays are the same in the two model series, although the 700 series has eliminated some test patterns as well as added a few. Table 2-3 lists the available screening test arrays grouped by type of screening pattern.

Table 2-4

THRESHOLD FIELD TEST PATTERNS FOR THE HFA II

Test Pattern	Point Density (°)	# Test Points	Typical Test Time (minutes per eye)
Central Tests			
Central 24-2	6	54	10 to 12
Central 30-2	6	76	12 to 15
Peripheral Tests			
Peripheral 60-4	12	60	12 to 15
Nasal step	†	14	2 to 3
Specialty Tests			
Central 10-2	2	68	10 to 12
Macula	2	161	8 to 10
Custom Tests			
Points can be added to any of the test patterns above or used alone			

† Test point density decreases with increasing eccentricity

Note that the central 166-point and the peripheral 68-point tests have been eliminated and the peripheral 60-point, full field 135 point, superior 36, and superior 64 tests have been added to the functionality of the HFA II models. Screening strategies are the same as in the earlier models, although the threshold-related strategy has been renamed the "two-zone strategy." Table 2-4 lists the threshold test patterns available. Note that the 24-1, 30-1, temporal crescent, neurological 20, and neurological 50 arrays are no longer available. Replacing the peripheral 30/60 arrays is the peripheral 60-4, which tests a group of points similar to the peripheral 30/60-2. SITA has been added as a strategy for the threshold tests but is not available for the macula or nasal step tests.

Esterman testing is available as a monocular or binocular test. Designed to assess disability due to loss of visual field, the Esterman tests incorporate a single-intensity strategy and use a 10 dB stimulus, testing 100 points in the monocular test and 120 points in the binocular test. The result is expressed as a percentage of the number of seen test points. These tests are selected from the specialty test menu.

Availability of tests may vary with the software version loaded on the instrument; the tests available on a particular machine can be found by touching the "show test library" button on the main menu screen. To view available tests, press the button for the class of test desired when the "choose a test type" window is displayed. As in the model 600 series, the user can define and save both custom screening and threshold tests for those situations where the standard battery of tests does not meet the particular need at hand. In addition, the main menu can be customized to reduce the time it takes to select and set up the instrument for the most commonly used tests.

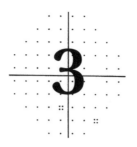

3

Setting Up a Perimetry System Using the Humphrey Field Analyzer

Introduction

Having a Humphrey Field Analyzer with all of its capabilities (as described in Chapter 2) is not sufficient to guarantee optimal visual field testing. Taking advantage of all the machine has to offer requires an integrated system for management of visual field information—ordering it, obtaining it, printing it out, storing it, retrieving it, interpreting it, and using it in the care of the patient. This chapter offers some suggestions for organizing a perimetry system around the Humphrey Field Analyzer in a manner that has proven useful for minimizing impediments to satisfactory perimetry and for maximizing the capabilities of the machine.

Useful results from automated perimetry depend heavily upon communication between all of the parties concerned—the health care provider (ie, the person who needs the information generated by the test), the technician (who has to administer the test and report the results back to the provider), and the patient (who must be informed about what is expected and be capable of performing properly). This communication forms a loop that goes from clinician to perimetrist to ensure the correct test is properly performed, and as feedback from perimetrist to clinician as a measure of patient performance. There must be a flow of information from the provider to the technician, technician to patient, patient to machine, and ultimately all back to the provider. Some suggestions for improving the flow of information will be discussed in Chapter 4. The location of the machine, the set-up of the system, and the operating procedures employed are all key components to be considered in order to obtain meaningful test results.

System Set-Up and Organization

Obtaining interpretable results with automated perimetry begins when a patient is scheduled for a visual field examination. The patient should be given a brief explanation about the nature of the test and what to expect during the examination. Performance can be enhanced with further education about the test by providing the patient with a hand-out that explains the exam upon the patient's arrival in the office. Patient information is covered in detail in Chapter 4. Figure 3-1 shows patient hand-outs in a chart box in the visual field waiting room of the authors' clinic. The medical record is placed in the box and the patient takes one

Figure 3-1. Patient instruction sheets.

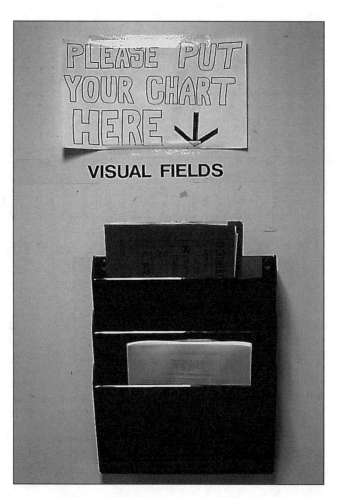

of the information hand-outs. The patient then has the opportunity to read the hand-out while the technician is setting up for the examination.

Machine Location

Automated perimetry is inherently difficult to perform comfortably and reliably. Tests may be long and tiring, and patients can easily become distracted, bored, or hypnotized. Therefore, the machine must be located in a place that is relatively free of noise or other sources of distraction. It should preferably be housed in its own room, which should have adequate ventilation and be of comfortable temperature. The testing room must be big enough to hold the machine, patients of varying size and shape, the technician, comfortable chairs for the patient and the technician, and should have storage facilities for floppy disks, printer ribbons, and paper. With the Humphrey Field Analyzer, it is not necessary that the room be dark since it operates under photopic conditions; however, the room lights should be capable of dimming. The machine should be positioned so as to avoid stray light on the bowl, not only from overhead lights but also from windows and doors, since any stray light may interfere with the patient's ability to detect the projected stimuli. The patient may respond to stray light thinking it was a projected stimulus, leading to false positive responses. Above all else, the patient's comfort and ability to concentrate on the task at hand are the main considerations in selecting a location for the machine. Figure 3-2 is a photograph of a perimetry room containing a Humphrey Field Analyzer. The room is six feet wide and eight feet long with the perimeter placed midway down the long wall on one side. The chairs are adjustable—adjusting the perimeter table and patient chair ensures that a patient can be positioned comfortably at the machine. Not seen in the photo is a small desk. Trial lenses and current disks are placed on the top of the desk. In the drawers are extra floppy disks, paper, printer ribbons, and other supplies. The lights are installed with dimmer switches, which allow the room to be darkened sufficiently for

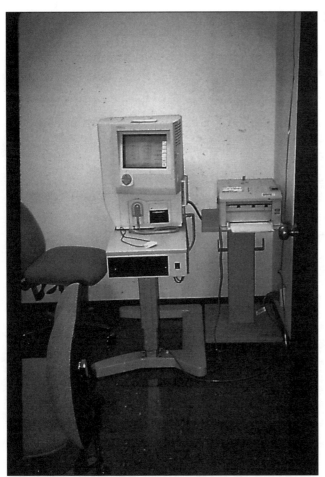

Figure 3-2. Visual field room with Humphrey perimeter.

the exam without making it difficult for the technician to find supplies. Prompts for the technician or instructions for the patient can be placed on the walls in the room. Figure 3-3 is a poster explaining fixation technique during foveal threshold determination. The poster serves as a reminder for the perimetrist in prompting the patient during the various initial stages of a test.

TECHNICIAN SPACE

The technician needs a place for recording and filing patient data, storing the perimeter manual for ready reference, and locating old visual fields stored on disk. In a practice where many visual fields are performed or where multiple machines may be in use at one time, it may be desirable to dedicate space for the technician outside the room where perimeters are used. In practices where fewer fields are performed, the technician can make use of space in the perimetry room. Figure 3-4 shows the technician desk in the authors' clinic. The boxes hold three by five-inch cards that contain visual field locator cards; these will be described in detail later in this chapter. The fan folder on the right contains visual field request forms for patients with visual field testing appointments. The request forms contain information the technician needs in order to perform the exam, including the type of test, strategy, and printout desired, the patient's refraction and phakic status, and follow-up information. The data needed by the technician to perform the test properly is discussed in Chapter 4.

Figure 3-3. Example of technician "prompts" taped to the wall of the examination room.

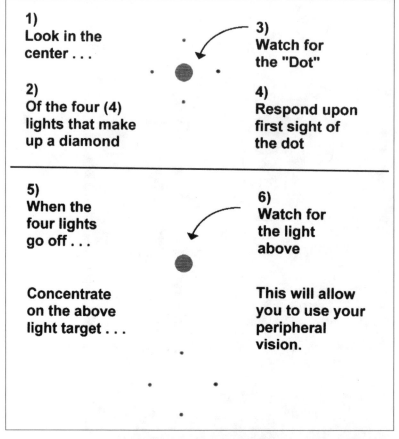

1)
Look in the center . . .

2)
Of the four (4) lights that make up a diamond

3)
Watch for the "Dot"

4)
Respond upon first sight of the dot

5)
When the four lights go off . . .

Concentrate on the above light target . . .

6)
Watch for the light above

This will allow you to use your peripheral vision.

Figure 3-4. Technician desk area in a dedicated perimetry space.

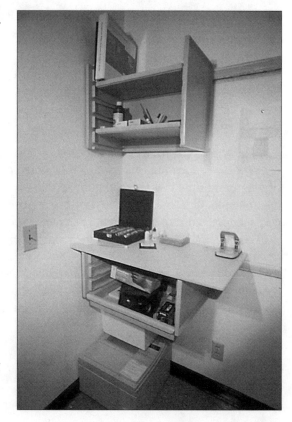

Patient Data Storage and Retrieval

Visual fields are stored digitally on magnetic media with the Humphrey perimeter. Large amounts of data can be stored in a relatively small amount of space: 200 visual field exams can fit on one 5¼-inch floppy disk, more on the 3½-inch floppies used with the HFA II. While this type of storage is highly reliable, data can be lost. Disk head crashes, accidental exposure to magnetic fields, and faulty diskettes, while not common occurrences, can lead to loss of visual fields. For this reason, multiple copies and frequent backing up of visual field data is vital. The recommended method of maintaining duplicate visual field data depends on the perimeter hardware. Dual floppy systems use one method while the hard-drive systems with a tape streamer use another.

Care should be taken when handling floppy disks. Static electricity and strong magnetic fields can ruin a disk. Keep the disks away from magnets and magnetic sources such as fluorescent light fixtures, audio speakers, and electrical appliances. Disks are fragile; avoid bending them or touching the media in the disk's exposed window. Do not write on the 5¼-inch disk with a pencil or a ballpoint pen, as this can damage the media inside. Instead, use a felt tip pen or write on the label before applying it to the disk. Avoid spilling liquids on the floppies as well. Store the floppy disks in their original boxes or in baskets or boxes specifically designed for their storage. Keep 5¼-inch disks in their paper jackets except when inserting them into the disk drive.

Floppy disks cannot be used for data storage straight out of the box; they must be prepared to receive data using a process called formatting. The disk format that Humphrey uses on the 600 series models is proprietary and different from that of other computer systems. Data on disks formatted for these Humphrey perimeters are not readable by Macintosh or IBM-type (DOS/Windows) personal computers (PCs) without additional software. Some software versions have an option to configure these Humphrey disks for STATPAC for Windows, a Microsoft Windows™ program designed to allow the clinician to perform further analysis of visual field data on a personal computer. STATPAC for Windows will be discussed in Chapter 9. The disk format used in the HFA II is the same as that used on IBM-compatible PCs; disks for these machines can be initialized on the field analyzer or on a compatible PC.

Formatting Diskettes on the HFA I

"Formatting a disk" is selected from the disk functions menu and takes several minutes to complete. Figure 3-5 shows the disk functions menu screen. The "initialize floppy disk" function option can be seen in the right-hand column of Figure 3-5. To format a floppy disk for use, the "hot spot" in the upper right-hand column next to "initialize floppy disk" is selected.

Formatting Diskettes on the HFA II

"Formatting a disk" on the HFA II is selected from the file functions menu. Figure 3-6 shows the file functions menu screen from the HFA II. To format a floppy disk for use, touch the button labeled "initialize floppy" at the bottom of the left-hand column.

DUAL FLOPPY DISK SYSTEMS

Many Humphrey Field Analyzers have two floppy disk drives; if your machine is equipped with a hard drive, this section does not apply.

Use of the Drives

Machines with two floppy disk drives should be used as follows: the top drive should be designated as the "chronological" drive. An initialized (formatted) disk is placed in this drive and stores all of the tests performed from the time it is first used until it is full (approximately 200 examinations). Chronological disks can be labeled in any manner you wish, such as CR1, CR2, etc. The label should also indicate the opening and closing dates for the disk.

Figure 3-5. Disk function screen of the Humphrey Field Analyzer.

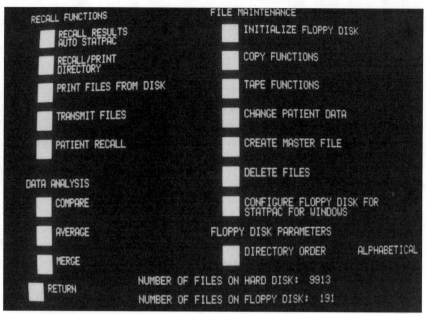

Figure 3-6. File functions menu screen from the Humphrey Field Analyzer II.

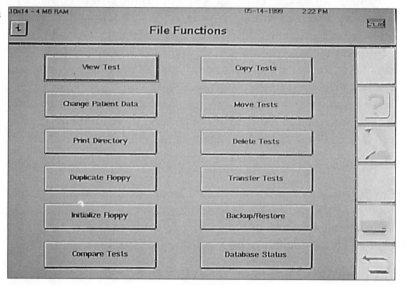

The bottom drive should be designated as the alphabetical drive. One floppy disk should be labeled with each letter of the alphabet, and the appropriate disk is inserted in the lower disk drive corresponding to the first letter of the patient's last name. Alphabetical disks should be labeled as A1, S3, etc, and each disk should be used until full. Again, include the opening and closing dates on the disk label, as is demonstrated in Figure 3-7.

Each time the Humphrey perimeter stores a visual field, it writes to both the upper and lower floppy disks. By using a chronological and alphabetical disk, data can easily be retrieved by date of test or patient name. Store the chronological disks in one box and the alphabetical disks in another. (For increased data safety, store the disks in different rooms as well.)

The HFA II model 730 has only a single 3½-inch disk drive. Be sure to back up the patient disks after each use or when full using the "duplicate floppy" button on the file functions screen. Store the duplicate set in a safe location separate from the working copies.

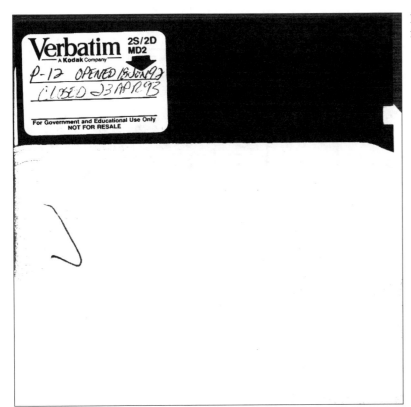

Figure 3-7. Sample patient data diskette from "alphabetical" drive.

Patient Visual Field Database

One of the greatest advantages of computerized perimetry is having quantitative data that the appropriate software can analyze for changes over time. An additional benefit is the ability to shorten testing procedures by using the results from prior tests as a starting point. However, in order to accomplish these things, the software must have access to the patient's previous examinations. If you are using a dual floppy disk system, you have to be able to locate the disks containing the previous patient data; if you are using more than one perimeter with hard drives, you must know which machine contains the desired fields. Thus, it is imperative to establish some sort of database for your patients. The essential information in the database should include the patient's name, test performed, stimulus size used, refraction used, and most importantly, the disks containing the patient's data. A well-organized system would allow follow-up testing even in the absence of the printout from the prior tests, whether or not the medical record is available.

With a floppy disk storage system in use and each patient's exams stored on two disks (an alphabetical and a chronological disk), for recall you must have a way of knowing on which disks this information is contained. How you organize your system will depend on how large you expect your perimetry system to be and what type of information management system you are comfortable dealing with. For smaller practices, you may wish to make an entry in the patient's medical record indicating where the results of the visual fields are stored or write the information directly on the printout of the field.

Card System

We have found an index card system to be useful and simple. A three by five-inch index card is filled out for each patient undergoing visual field testing. One side of the card contains identifying data, including name, social security number, date of birth, address, and telephone number. On the other side, an entry is made for each examination that includes the test performed, date of the exam, stimulus size used, refraction used, and the disks upon which the examination results are stored, as seen in Figure 3-8. When the patient returns for a follow-up examination, the card is pulled and the alphabetical disk containing the previous examinations is used (provided the disk is not full); the chronological disk serves as the back-up in case the data cannot be located on the alphabetical disk. For performing STATPAC analyses (see Chapter 5), all data

Figure 3-8. Back side of an index card from the patient visual field database.

DATE	TYPE TEST	DISK #	STIM SIZE	Rx USED
Nov 87	30-2 su	H-4	III	+2.25 -2.50 x 097
16 Feb 90	30-2	H-10	II	+2.00 -1.00 x 094 +3.00
10-7-91	30-2	H-14	III	+3.00
9 Oct 92	30-2	H-17 HD	III	+3.25 -1.50 x 078 HD +3.25 -1.75 x 093 #1
21 Jan 94	30-2	H-19 HD	III	+4.00 -1.25 x 100 +3.25 -1.25 x 085
21 Dec 94	30-2	HD #1	II	+3.00 -1.25 x 080 +1.25 SPH
27 Oct 77	24-2	#1	III	+3.00 -1.50 x 077 +3.50
27 Feb 97	24-2	#2	III	+3.00 -2.00 x 090

must be on one disk; if the patient's tests are on different disks, each file must be copied to a single disk. Keep a "trash" disk near the perimeter for this purpose.

Computerized Relational Database

An alternative to keeping a card file is to place the database on an office or personal computer. Any database program, such as DBASE III+™ (Ashton-Tate, 1985, 1986) or Microsoft Access™ (Microsoft, 1995, 1997) can be used. A computer database is much like a card file. Each record in a database is like a single card in the card file, with each field in the database corresponding to an entry on the card. Computer databases are generally referred to as "flat" or "relational." Using the card file analogy, a flat database contains records in which each card represents a single visual field examination. Patients with multiple visual field examinations would have multiple cards in the card file. In a relational database, information such as a patient's name and phone number would be stored only once; records with the patient's demographic data would include a unique value that would be related to records containing visual field data, such as what test was performed, when it was performed, and on what disk the field can be found. Using relational databases allows more flexibility in the design of the database and in later modifications to it, but either type can satisfy the needs for visual field record keeping.

Whatever type of database structure is used, the basic information required is the same as is used on the card file system described above. The advantage of a computerized database is that information can be easily located. This can provide a means for quality improvement in a practice and be used in outcome analysis. For example, a practitioner might want to determine if the information obtained from central 30-2 threshold tests was any more useful in his or her practice than that from central 24-2 exams. The database could be queried to list the most recent 30 of each of those types of visual fields. The fields could be printed out and compared. It is easy to add additional database fields of interest. For example, a field could be added that corresponds to progression of visual field defects (improved, stable, or worse). The database could be queried to find all fields showing deterioration in a group of glaucoma patients and that information used to evaluate the effectiveness of therapy. There are a number of commercially available database software programs; selection of a program, designing the visual field database with it, and implementing its use in a clinical practice is beyond the scope of this text and is left to the individual practitioner.

Humphrey Hard Drive/Streamer Tape Systems

Description

The hard disk on models so equipped can store 33,000 or more visual fields, depending on the hard disk size. This large storage capacity will last the life of the instrument in most practices. Since data can be lost from hard disks, frequent backing up is necessary for safety in the event of a catastrophic disk crash. The tape streamer can easily store all of the data contained on the hard drive, but backing up to the streamer is time consuming (backing up 5,000 fields takes about 45 minutes) and not a practical method of back-up during the day while the instrument is in use. A chronological disk, as described in the section on dual floppy disk systems, should be used in addition to the hard drive. Again, as each chronological disk is filled, it should be closed and a new chronological disk opened. You will thus have two copies of each field, plus the back-up on tape.

Tape back-ups should be performed at the end of the day or at least on a weekly basis. In the event of loss of data from the hard disk, the tape can be used to restore data from the most recent back-up once the hardware problem has been fixed. The chronological disk can then be used to copy the fields performed since the last tape back-up to restore all of the fields onto the hard disk. Disk copying functions and tape back-up are selected from the "disk functions" menu. Refer to the manual for restoring data from the tape to the hard disk.

Database Functions of the Hard Drive

Perimeters equipped with a hard drive have a built-in database system that is proprietary to Humphrey. Tests are sorted alphabetically by the patients' names but may also be viewed in a chronological sort. All disk functions that require patient names can use the name search function, allowing the technician to select the desired patient from a list, unless of course, the patient has not yet had a visual field test performed. Selecting from a pick list helps to ensure that no patient is entered with multiple names (Smith, A and Smith,A [different spacing] are seen by the perimeter as two different patient names, for example). To find a file on the hard disk, the disk must be selected after choosing the function desired (eg, printing files from a disk). A keyboard is displayed on the screen with prompts to enter all or part of the desired patient's name using the light pen. Once entered, a list of names and examinations will appear. Scroll up or down as necessary and select the file(s) desired. The database can also be used as a starting point to enter patient data before beginning a new examination on a patient previously tested. After selecting "enter new patient data," the menu screen displays a hot box in the lower right-hand corner labeled "enter patient data from disk files." When this is selected, the screen keyboard is displayed and the patient's name can be entered. With this feature, only the data that has changed (eg, refraction or pupil size) needs to be entered. Testing proceeds as usual after entering the patient data.

On the HFA II models equipped with hard drives, choose "recall patient data" from the "patient data 1" screen. Select the source (hard drive or floppy), then "proceed." Use the scroll buttons to locate the desired patient. Touch the screen over the patient's name to select it, then touch the "proceed" button. The selected patient's information can be added to or modified as needed.

A clinical practice with one Humphrey perimeter equipped with a hard drive can function without any other database system. Practices with two or more machines with hard drives require some method of knowing on which hard drive a patient's previous visual fields are located. Several methods can meet this requirement. A simple method is to make a notation in the patient's chart. This works well when records are always available, but may not work in multispecialty practices where charts are not always immediately available. Looking up a patient on the hard drive also works, but this method can lead to long waiting times if a patient's fields are located on a machine already in use. A third method is to use a card system, such as that described in the dual floppy drives section. If a patient's fields are on the hard drive of a machine in use, the fields can be copied from the floppy disks that also exist. A fourth method is to copy all the fields performed during the day from each perimeter's chronological disk to the hard drive of all the other perimeters at the end of each day. Using this method, the hard drives on each perimeter have the same database at the beginning of each day. Fewer total fields can be stored, however. Since the hard drive can contain about 33,000 fields, if each perimeter has the same database, only 33,000 fields can be stored; if the perimeters do not contain common patients, 33,000 fields per machine can be stored.

Humphrey perimeters equipped with dual floppy drives can be upgraded to the hard drive system. Contact your Humphrey service representative for additional information and pricing.

Patient Recall

For disease processes known to affect the visual field in a progressive manner, follow-up examinations at appropriate intervals are essential. The Humphrey 600 series perimeters have a feature that permits you to print a list containing names of patients who have not had visual fields performed in a specified time limit. While the default range is six to 24 months, the range can be changed, as long as the oldest field is no more than 24 months old. This patient recall function is available on dual floppy disk systems, but it is most useful when all exams are stored in one location (ie, the hard drive). The perimeter can "remember" the names on previous patient recall lists. There is an option to print all names that fall within the specified time limit or just the names that have not appeared on previous lists.

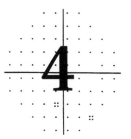

Testing the Patient

Introduction

Before the development of automated perimetry, visual field testing was as difficult for the test administrator as for the test taker. Automation has simplified the process by removing the boring, tedious, mechanical aspects of the test (monitoring fixation, recording responses, selecting the appropriate stimuli, moving the target, drawing the plots, etc) but has not eliminated other very important functions of the perimetrist. There are many aspects of the test situation that are controllable by the perimetrist, which, if optimized, increase the chances for obtaining reliable useful results.

The object of visual field testing is to obtain visual field data that is reliable, accurate, and representative (to the best of the machine's ability) of the true state of the island of vision as it exists at the time the test is done in order to provide the clinician with the information necessary for appropriate patient care. Since visual field testing is a "psychophysiologic" function (implying that factors other than the patient's actual visual field are responsible for what appears on the printout), it should be possible through proper understanding of the test options by the clinician, of the test procedures by the patient, and of the operation of the machine and the perimetry system by the perimetrist, to minimize the effect of "human factors" and obtain meaningful results. This chapter describes how to select and administer a visual field test to a patient using the Humphrey Field Analyzer in a way that maximizes the results, making the test as easy as possible for the patient while providing the clinician with the desired information.

Test Selection and Ordering

It is the job of the clinician to know what information is desired from the visual field test, what the test options are, and which ones to use to obtain the desired information. It is not the job of the perimetrist (unless the perimetrist is the clinician) to decide, having been told to "do a visual field test," which test to administer and how to administer it. The technician controls the test situation and must make decisions regarding the test procedures with regard to the patient's adaptation to the test. Appropriate adjustments must be made as the test proceeds. The role of the technician as test administrator will be explained later in this chapter. Please remember that some of the test grids and strategies discussed in this chapter may not be available on all models of the instrument or in all versions of the software, although each machine should have something similar.

When the Humphrey Field Analyzer first appeared on the market, it was criticized as offering "too many tests," making test selection somewhat bewildering. At face value this may be a valid criticism, given the large number of test arrays and various strategies available. With the ability to create a user-defined menu, the number of test options can be pared down to include only those that are frequently used. It is recommended that the clinician review the available tests and strategies and set up the user-defined menu to meet the needs of the particular practice setting. Most practitioners will find four or five examination options apply to the vast majority of clinical situations. Table 4-1 lists the types of patients commonly encountered in clinical practice and recommendations for appropriate tests for those patients. Note that "routine" visual field testing is not recommended. That would be like ordering neuro-imaging for everyone with a headache—the yield of pathologic results would be too low to justify the costs. Automated perimetry should be used as an adjunctive test for the diagnosis and management of conditions known to affect the visual field and not as part of a routine eye examination of a patient with no relevant complaints. It is appropriate to proceed with automated perimetry when a gross screening test such as confrontation visual field testing suggests a defect.

If screening tests are to be used, remember that the obtainable information is limited. For example, the field shown in Figure 4-1 is clinically useless. The few nasal misses and the two in the temporal field do not give the clinician any information upon which to base a diagnosis. This patient must be tested again with a more quantified test.

Figure 4-2 is an example of a threshold-related screen obtained from an elderly woman with limited capacity for the test procedures. Most of the points in the superior hemifield were missed at six decibels brighter than expected normal. The pattern is suggestive of a superior altitudinal defect. It can be inferred that this is a very disturbed field since the patient required a stimulus size V and the central reference level was 30 dB. Still, it is not known what the magnitude of the loss is in the superior field: it could be anywhere from seven decibels up to absolute. Additional information can be obtained by using the three-zone strategy, as illustrated in Figure 4-3. Here, points not seen at six decibels brighter than expected are tested with the maximum stimulus intensity. Points perceiving the maximum stimulus are labeled with the "X," indicating that they are relative defects, while those not seen at 10,000 asb are labeled with the black square. The magnitude of the relative defects is not known. Worsening of the field over time can only be detected if the number of absolute defects increases at the expense of the relative defects. Therefore, if screening tests are to be used at all, it is recommended that the quantify defects strategy be used whenever possible. An example is given in Figure 4-4. Here, each point missed on the initial screen has threshold determined and the printout shows the difference between the measured threshold and expected value. The resultant defect depths can be followed over time for improvement or worsening. Although not as effective as a threshold test, at least the quantify defects strategy of a screen offers some useful information.

The patient whose threshold-related 120-point screen is shown in Figure 4-5 presented with a two-day history of headache and blurred vision. The visual field was obtained because of a detectable defect on the right side on confrontation testing. The screening test revealed multiple misses on the right side of the visual field, suggestive of a right homonymous hemianopsia, mostly involving the inferior quadrant. The pattern of missed spots is suggestive of a posterior pathway lesion since the pattern is congruous. The patient underwent threshold testing 26 days later, shown in Figure 4-6. Undoubtedly there has been some improvement in the field, but since the first field was not quantified, it is difficult to know how much improvement occurred. The loss pattern is highly congruous and localizes a cerebral vascular accident posterior to the occipital cortex. The 30-2 test in this case is more informative than the screen.

The final aspect of test selection is knowing what you are looking for. For example, the 120-point full field screening test, as shown in Figures 4-3 to 4-5, offers a tight array of points straddling the vertical midline and is suited to testing patients with suspected neurological defects expected to localize to either side of the vertical. The 76-point screen is the same pattern of points as the 30-2 threshold test and may be a good "training" test for a glaucoma patient's indoctrination into automated perimetry. Sometimes, however, a clinician knows exactly what he or she wants to find and picks the specific test pattern to detect it.

Table 4-1

SUGGESTIONS FOR TEST SELECTION

Type of Patient	Test Type	Array	Strategy	Stimulus Size	Follow-up
Routine examination, no complaints	Visual field testing not recommended	n/a	n/a	n/a	n/a
Complains of loss "side vision"	Screen	120 point	Three zone or quantify defects	III	Threshold of testing
Complains of "spots" in central vision	Amsler grid	n/a	n/a	n/a	n/a
	Threshold	30-2, 10-2	Full threshold or SITA	III	Overview, change analysis
Glaucoma suspect/ ocular hypertension	24-2, 30-2	III	Full threshold, SITA, or SWAP (V for SWAP)	III	overview, Change analysis
Glaucoma—early moderate	Threshold	30-2, 24-2	Full threshold or SITA	III	Glaucoma to change probability*
Glaucoma—advanced	Threshold	30-2, 24-2	Full threshold or SITA	III, IV	Glaucoma change probability*
Glaucoma—end stage	Threshold	30-2, 24-2	Full threshold or SITA	V	Stimulus V overview
	Threshold	10-2	Full threshold or SITA	III	Overview, change analysis
Neurologic: detection, asymptomatic patient	Screen	120 point	Quantify defects	III	Threshold test
Neurologic: detection, symptomatic patient	Threshold	30-2	Full threshold or SITA	III	Overview, change analysis
Neurologic: patient requiring serial examinations	Threshold	30-2	Full threshold or SITA	III	Overview, change analysis
Patients with Amsler grid defects	Threshold	10-2	Full threshold or SITA	III	Overview, change analysis
Monitoring patients at risk for maculopathy (eg, drug toxicity)	Threshold	10-2	Full threshold or SITA	III white, red	Overview, change analysis
Any patient having difficulty with threshold test	Threshold	24-2	FASTPAC or SITA	III	Overview, change analysis
	Screen	76 point	Quantify defects	III	None available can try threshold test next time
Frail, infirm, disabled patients	Screen	76 point	Threshold related, three-zone	III	None available

*Not yet available for SITA or SWAP

Figure 4-1. A threshold-related screening test.

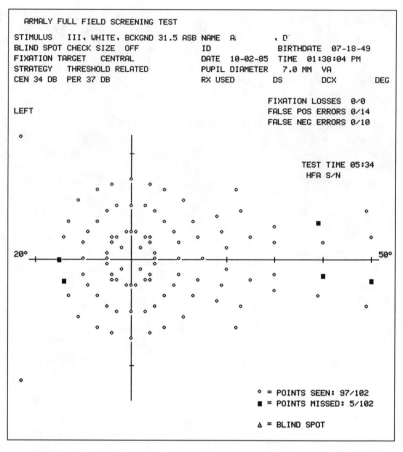

Figure 4-2. Seventy-six-point threshold-related screening test performed because the patient was physically incapable of performing any other type of test.

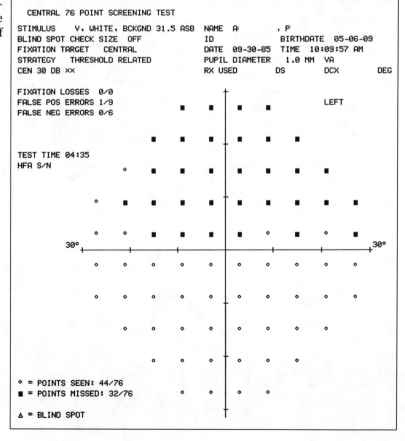

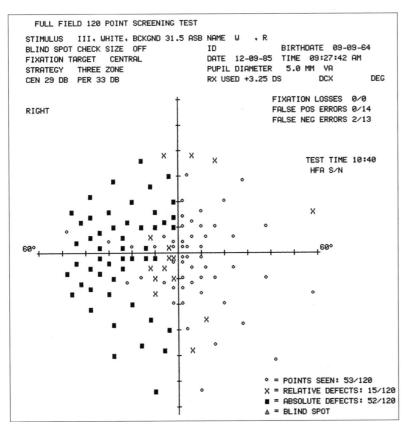

Figure 4-3. The three-zone screening test.

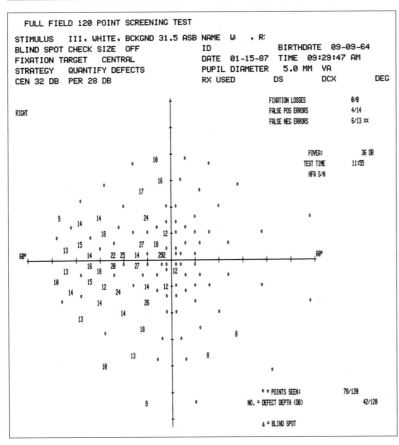

Figure 4-4. A screening test performed with the quantify defects strategy.

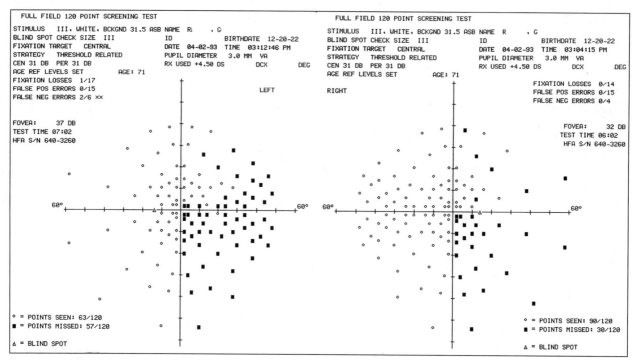

Figure 4-5. An incongruous right homonymous hemianopic defect detected on a 120-point screening test with the threshold-related strategy.

The patient shown in Figure 4-7 was seen in consultation for glaucoma and had prior Goldmann fields demonstrating a dense superior arcuate scotoma. Her optic nerve was missing rim tissue at the six o'clock position, consistent with the Goldmann field. The 30-2 test revealed only mild disturbances in the superior hemifield. Suspecting that the scotoma was missed, the test was repeated with the 30-1, shown in Figure 4-8. The scotoma was found, lurking between the test points of the 30-2.

Patients with end-stage disease pose difficult problems for follow-up testing, since there may not be enough visual field remaining to provide data to follow. One such patient is shown in Figure 4-9. The entire field is significantly depressed and no diagnostic pattern of focal loss is discernable. Such patients should be tested with larger test objects, such as the stimulus V. Using the larger stimulus increases the range of sensitivity by up to seven decibels and "amplifies" the remaining field. By testing the patient in Figure 4-7 with a stimulus V, the double-arcuate nature of the loss is more apparent. The resultant field is shown in Figure 4-10 .

Finally, the remaining bastions of sensitivity in this field can be elucidated by use of the central 10-2 test. This grid, with 2° spacing, can show exactly what is left in the central field and can be followed for worsening that may not be apparent in the wider-spaced grid. Figure 4-11 shows the remaining central field of the patient in Figures 4-9 and 4-10.

Once the decision to perform a visual field test has been made, the test to be used is selected, and the parameters of the test are decided; the necessary information must be communicated to the person who will administer the test. The essential information includes how soon it is to be done, when the patient will be seen again, what test is to be done, how the test is to be done (strategy), what type of printouts and analysis are required, the distance refraction, dilate the pupils or not, and what stimulus to use (size and color). The way this information is communicated will vary with the complexity of the practice setting. A solo practitioner, maintaining the records of the practice on the premises, will be able to schedule the test and include the relevant information in the medical record. The record can then be made available to the perimetrist when the patient comes in for the examination.

A multiprovider practice offers more difficulty. Communication may still be via the medical record, but the ensurance of proper follow-up becomes the issue. Difficulties arise in practice situations in which the

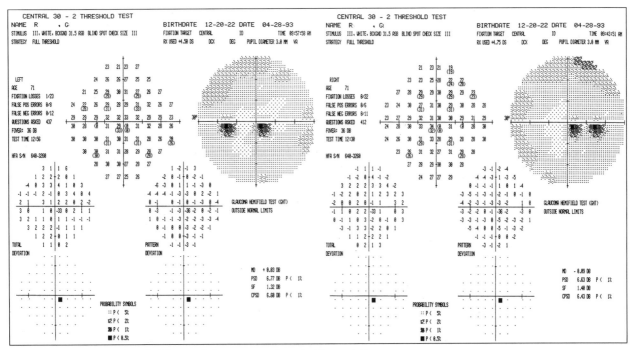

Figure 4-6. The 30-2 threshold test of the same patient in Figure 4-5.

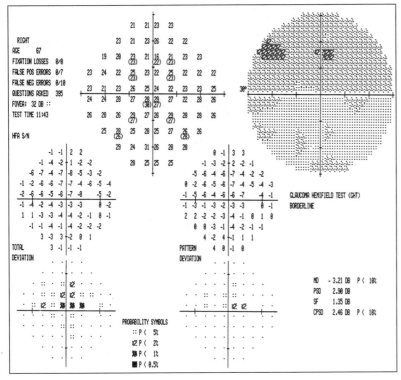

Figure 4-7. A 30-2 threshold test performed in a patient known to have a superior arcuate scotoma on Goldmann testing and missing rim tissue at the inferior pole of the disc.

records are not maintained on the premises, such as large health maintenance organizations, Veteran's Administration hospitals, military hospitals, large multispecialty groups employing a single record for each patient, which include all specialties within the organization, etc. Visual field ordering information contained in a medical record that has the potential for not being available at the time the test is administered is the same as having no information at all. The technician then does not know what test to administer, how to manage the pupils, or which correcting lens to use. The technician should not rely on reading the glasses the patient is wearing to determine the correcting lens, since patients may show up for the test without them ("I

Figure 4-8. A 30-1 test from the same patient as in Figure 4-7, which found the missing scotoma.

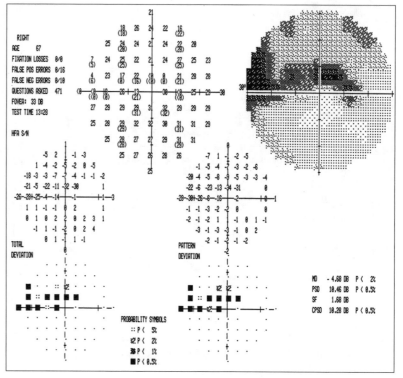

Figure 4-9. Advanced loss in a patient with severe optic nerve damage. The nature of the loss cannot be discerned because of the diffuse depression.

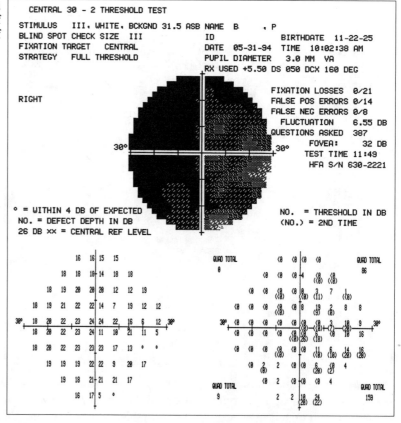

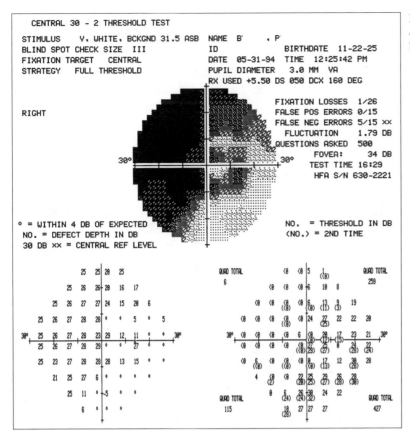

Figure 4-10. The same patient as in Figure 4-9 tested with a stimulus size V. The double arcuate nature of the loss is revealed.

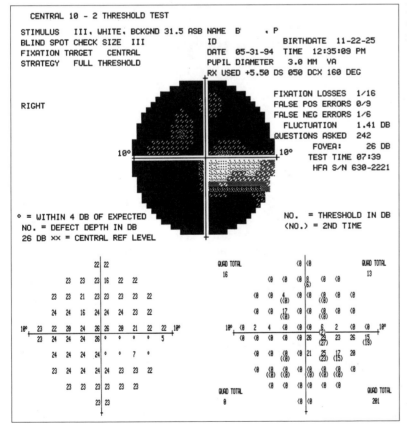

Figure 4-11. The remaining central island of vision in the patient from Figure 4-9, as mapped by the 10-2 test.

left them in the car"), or the prescription may have been changed and the new glasses have not yet been picked up. A proposed solution to avoiding the possibility of miscommunication is to use a visual field ordering form, such as the one shown in Figure 4-12. The form is filled out when the decision to order a visual field is made. The provider indicates which type of field is desired (Humphrey or Goldmann), the date of the order, when the test should be done (allowing for advance scheduling to coincide with the next visit), and when the patient is to be seen again. The option of seeing the patient on the same day of the exam before the test is done is usually to allow a recheck of the refraction. Patients requiring pupillary dilation for the visual field test are also seen before the test, allowing for pressure checks, dilation, determination of the refraction once dilated, and fundus exam (reducing patient visits). An alternative for patients requiring dilation for the examination is to perform a dilated examination and refraction at the time of the visit at which the visual field is ordered and indicate on the ordering form what the dilated refraction is, circle "dilated" next to the specified distance refraction, and indicate specific dilating instructions for the perimetrist. Systems with multiple providers and locations can indicate who ordered the test and from which site. The test, options, and print-out(s) desired are selected, and the specific test instructions indicated (refraction, stimulus size and color, dilation instructions). The perimetrist must be made aware of the patients lacking accommodation; therefore, the form allows for the identification of those patients who are aphakic, pseudophakic, or who have been dilated. The form also allows for the identification of patients who will be tested while wearing their own contact lenses. Alerting the perimetrist to this prevents the use of unnecessary additional distance correction. Once the form has been completed, it is brought to the scheduling desk for appointment. The date and time of the appointment are noted on the top of the form, and the form is then forwarded to the visual field testing area, where it is kept on file. When the patient reports for the examination, the form is pulled and all necessary information is then available, whether or not the chart has arrived or if the patient remembered to bring his/her eyeglasses. The bottom portion of the form allows for the technician to comment on test performance, which is useful information to have when interpreting the results of the test. Visual field interpretation is discussed in detail in Chapter 5.

Setting Up the Machine For an Examination

STEP 1: GATHER THE NECESSARY INFORMATION

The Humphrey Field Analyzer must be set up for each examination prior to the start of testing. Organization of the testing area and methods for storing patient demographic information have been discussed in Chapter 3. The technician needs the visual field ordering information and patient information to proceed with machine set-up. In the authors' system, the ordering information is found on the visual field order form, and the patient information is found on a yellow index card (previously described). Using the information in the patient database, locate any disks containing data for the patient being tested. Place the most recent alphabetical disk into the floppy drive. If the patient has information on more than one disk and you are not using the hard drive system, you will want to copy all of the patient's prior data onto one floppy disk for analysis of changes over time. If you have a hard drive system, make sure all of the patient's prior fields are present. Copy any fields present on floppy disks to the hard drive.

STEP 2: IDENTIFY THE PATIENT TO THE MACHINE

The patient's name, identification number (social security number is recommended as a unique identifier), and birth date are entered using the light pen and the cathode ray tube (CRT) display on the 600 series models, or using the touch screen CRT display or keyboard on the HFA II models. It is important to enter the patient's name exactly as it was entered on any prior examinations, since any alteration will cause the machine to fail to find all of the patient's examinations for overview, change, or STATPAC analysis. Joe Smith, Joseph Smith, and Joe E. Smith are all different patients as far as the machine is concerned (see

date scheduled: _____
time scheduled: _____

Visual Field Order Form

[] Humphrey   [] Goldmann

telephone: _____

ADDRESSOGRAPH STAMP

Instructions for using this form: All **required** information indicated in
bold. No test will be scheduled if this information is not supplied. Indicate choices by circling when choices are listed or by
placing check marks in appropriate spaces.

date exam ordered: _____
date exam desired: __ routine in ___ month(s) / week(s)   __add-on ASAP
                          __ today (emergency)   __other (specify exact date) _____
next appointment with provider:
     __ same day as field (before / after)
     __ anytime after field within _____ week(s) / month(s)

provider: _____ location: NMCSD ophth / NMCSD optom / region

Test desired: Threshold: 30-2 / 24-2 / 10-2 Strategy: full threshold / FASTPAC / SITA / SWAP
     __ other threshold test (specify) _____
     __ 120 point screen   Strategy: threshold related / three-zone / quantify defects
     __ other screening test (and strategy) _____
     __ Goldmann: screening / glaucoma / neurological

Printout for threshold tests (if other than standard STATPAC single field analysis):
     __ value table / graytone / defect depth / triple (includes all three formats)
     __ profile (specify cut) _____
     __ compare with last visual field
     __ glaucoma change probability   Prior visual field here? [] yes   [] no
     __ overview / change analysis

distance refraction: OD   _____-_____x_____ aphakic / dilated / contacts
                            OS   _____-_____x_____ aphakic / dilated / contacts

     __ non-standard stimulus size (default = III): ___ OD ___ OS
     __ non-standard stimulus color (default = white): red / blue / green

(Technician note: dilated or aphakic patients require full add. All others, including contact lens patients, require appropriate
add for age as specified in the manual.)

Technician comments: Patient understood test?   yes / no
                             Required constant supervision?   yes / no
                             Exhibited good fixation behavior?   yes / no
                             Complained?   yes / no
                             Rested frequently?   yes / no
                             Required larger stimulus than ordered? yes / no

Other comments/observations: _____
_____
_____
(At completion of exam, attach this form to printout) **tech initial:** _____

Figure 4-12. A visual field ordering form.

Figure 4-13. Test performed with the incorrect birth date. Note the nonsignificant mean deviation.

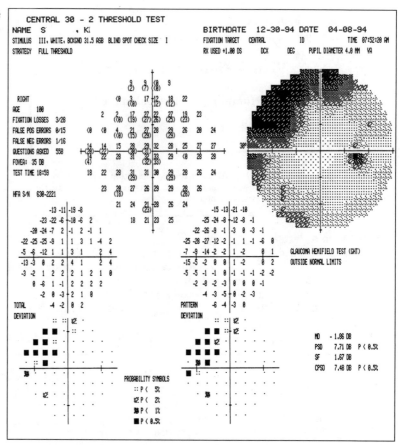

Chapter 3 for additional information about patient data). Entering the correct birth date is essential for proper calculation of the add if the automatic trial lens calculation feature is used and to tell STATPAC how old the patient is for comparison to the correct age-matched normal population. Figure 4-13 is an example of a test performed with the patient's birth date entered with the correct month and day, but with the present year entered in lieu of the correct year. The machine does not recognize that the birth date entered for the examination is after the date of the exam! It does recognize the year and assumes that it is 1894, thus making the patient 100 years old. The patient is then compared to an age-matched population of 100-year-olds and appears to have a mean deviation of -1.86 dB (mean deviation is discussed in Chapter 5). In reality, the patient was born in 1954, and the printout with the correct birth date appears in Figure 4-14. Compared to 40-year-olds, the mean deviation is -6.51. Comparing a patient to an older population will make the deviations appear smaller since the comparison threshold values are lower, thus care must be taken when entering the patient information in the machine. The later versions of the operating software for the perimeter allow the technician to recall patient data from disk files. This options assures that there will be no variations in the patient's name or birth date. The 700 series models are all compatible with years beginning with 20 (ie, it is "Y2K" compliant). A software fix is available for the 600 series so that there will not be a problem calculating the patients' ages once the year changes to 2000 and greater. This involves an EPROM change. Contact your Humphrey representative for more information.

STEP 3: SELECT THE CORRECTING LENS

Since a visual field test requires the patient to discern an often faint test object against a lighted background, chances of the patient seeing the stimulus are increased if the stimulus is in focus. The Humphrey Field Analyzer 600 series models use a bowl of 33 cm radius, therefore the patient must be optically corrected for one-third of a meter. The HFA II models use a radius of 30 cm. The machine provides a lens holder into which the operator inserts the appropriate lens based on the distance refraction. The distance refrac-

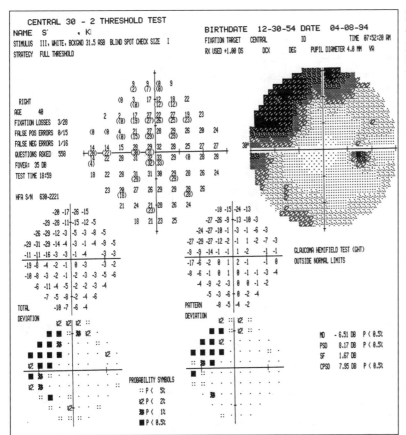

Figure 4-14. Same examination as Figure 4-13 with the correct birth date. The patient is now compared to the appropriate age-corrected normals. Mean deviation is now highly significant.

tion used should be recent and appropriate to the test situation. Ideally, visual acuity should be checked with the refraction to be used to assure that the acuity is at its known best. If not, and the acuity improves with a pinhole, the patient will need to be refracted prior to performing the visual field. All patients undergoing dilation for the visual field test must have their refraction checked post-dilation, either just prior to the visual field test or at a recent previous visit. Once the distance refraction is established, the lens to be used is calculated in one of two ways.

The simplest method is by using the machine's automatic lens calculation feature. The following steps are used in revision 9.3 of the operating software on the HFA 700 series. Check the manual for instructions for your version of instrument and software. From the main or user-defined menu, select "enter new patient data." Enter all of the information, particularly the birth date (taking the precautions discussed above to enter the correct birth year). Select "rx used" and enter the sphere, cylinder, and axis for the right and left eyes using the column headed "distance rx." Select "calculate trial lens using distance rx and birth date," and the machine will determine the lens to be used for the test based on the distance rx and the appropriate add for the age of the patient calculated from the birth date you entered. Obviously, the clock in the machine must be set to the correct date for the calculation to be performed correctly. The date and time appear on the top of the patient data entry screen and should be verified as correct prior to proceeding. After selecting the "calculate" button, the trial lens to be used will appear in the left-hand column headed "trial lens" and on the patient data screen next to the "rx used" button. The "rx used" information will appear on the printouts as well.

The alternative method to determine the lens to be used and the only method for software versions not offering the automatic calculation feature is to manually calculate the lens based on the distance rx and the patient's age. Table 4-2 summarizes the steps used for selecting the trial lens. The small insert table showing the age-specific adds should be copied and taped to the side of the field analyzer or to the trial lens set for ready reference. Remember to use the add as specified by the manufacturer, not the add found in the patient's glasses. Often patients read at distances greater than one-third of a meter and will not be corrected for the

Table 4-2

DETERMINING THE CORRECTING LENS

1. Ignore cylinder powers of less than 0.25 diopters. Calculate spherical equivalent power for lenses with cylinder between 0.25 and 1.50 diopters (to calculate spherical equivalent power, add half the cylinder power to that of the sphere, then ignore the cylinder). Use the full cylinder for cylinders greater than 1.50 diopters. This determines the resultant lens.

2. Determine the add required based on age or accommodation from the chart:

Patient's Age	Add Needed
< 30	no add
30 - 39	+1.00
40 - 44	+1.50
45 - 49	+2.00
50 - 54	+2.50
> 55	+3.00

Aphakic, pseudophakic, or dilated (any age): +3.00

3. Add the resultant distance lens to the age-required add. This is the lens to be used.

Table 4-3

EXAMPLES OF TRIAL LENS CALCULATION

Patient's Age	Distance Rx	Cylinder Action	Resultant Rx	Accommodative State	Add Based on Age or Accommodation	Lens Used for Test
29	-1.75-0.25 x 175	Ignore	-1.75 sph	Normal	+0.00	-1.75 sph
32	-1.75-1.00 x 145	Add 1/2 to sph	-2.25 sph	Normal	+1.00	-1.25 sph
54	+2.25-2.00 x 090	Use full	+2.25-2.00 x 090	Normal	+2.50	+4.75-2.00 x 090
52, on pilo	-1.00-3.00 x 105	Use full	-1.00-3.00 x 105	Dilated for exam = none	+3.00	+2.00-3.00 x 105
72	+4.00-1.00 x 085	Add 1/2 to sph	+3.50 sph	Normal	+3.00	+6.50 sph
53 pseudophake	+2.00-4.00 x 070	Use full	+2.00-4.00 x 070	Pseudophakic = none	+3.00	+5.00-4.00 x 070

distance of the visual field test with the add in their glasses. Don't forget to perform the trial lens calculations for each eye separately. Table 4-3 gives a few examples of trial lens calculations.

Once the correcting lens has been determined, insert the lenses into the lens holder with the sphere in the slot closest to the patient and the cylinder, oriented with the correct axis, in the far slot. Make sure the lenses used are the rimless variety, as ordinary trial lenses such as those found in most examination lanes have thick black rims that will block out a portion of the patient's visual field, leading to artifactual loss. The correcting lens must be removed when testing any portion of the visual field outside of the central 30°. The machine will pause when testing of the central 30° is completed and will prompt the technician to remove the lens prior to proceeding with the peripheral field. Figure 4-15 is an example of a patient tested with the correct distance lens, however, the operator forgot to use the necessary add. The patient was undercorrected at the test distance by +3.00 diopters and was thus out of focus, resulting in a field showing diffuse loss of sensitivity. The effect of incorrect lenses will be discussed further in Chapter 5. Patients should be encouraged to advise the technician if the interior of the machine seems out of focus so that appropriate adjustments can be made.

STEP 4: SELECT THE TEST TO BE USED

The visual field ordering sheet or the medical record should contain all of the test parameters desired by the clinician. These include the type of test (threshold versus screening), the array of points, the test strate-

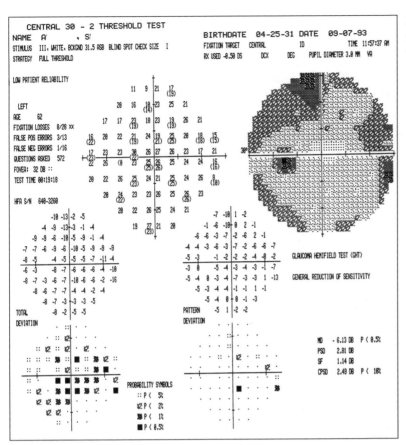

Figure 4-15. Patient tested with correct distance lens but no add. Note diffuse loss of sensitivity.

gy, and stimulus size and color. Select the appropriate options from the menus. Nonstandard parameters, such as the requirement to test with a stimulus other than the default size III, may require selection from the "change parameters" screen. The fluctuation test and determination of foveal threshold may also need to be configured in some versions of the operating software. Make sure the machine is configured to perform the test as ordered by the requester. The machine should now be ready for the patient. Remember that frequently used configurations and set-ups can be added to the user-defined menu so that it will not be necessary to go through all of the above steps to set up the machine each time a patient is tested.

Patient Set-Up

PATIENT INSTRUCTIONS

While the machine is being set up, the patient should have the opportunity to become familiar with the test procedures. A printed information sheet is most helpful for preparing the patient for the experience of automated visual field testing. One such information sheet is shown in Figure 4-16. Patients tend to be anxious while undergoing medical procedures, and this may be especially true when the procedure is unfamiliar and foreign. The patient may have been told that he or she has been scheduled for a test but not have any idea what it is about. Maximizing the patient's understanding of the procedure, what it is for, how it is performed, what he or she is supposed to do, and what to expect during the test can all help to reduce the apprehension that can impede performance. It is especially important to tell patients in advance that there will be periods of time during the test when the lights will be too dim to be seen as the machine attempts to determine "how sensitive" their eyes are. This helps reduce the feeling that they must be blind when they can't see the light. Another important point to emphasize is that they have the ability to rest when needed by holding down the

---

Visual Field Testing -- Information for Patients

Your doctor has ordered a visual field examination for you. This test determines the sensitivity of your peripheral vision, that is, how well you see "out of the corner of your eye." The examination will be performed by a computerized machine known as the Humphrey Field Analyzer, which is amongst the most advanced methods available today for measuring the visual field. The examination is not difficult, but there are some aspects of it with which you should be familiar. Please read this material prior to your examination.

Since this is an examination of your "side" vision, it is most important that you hold your eye still and look straight ahead at all times. Inside the machine there is a steady yellow light for you to look at. Unless instructed otherwise, you should stare at this light at all times. The test lights will flash on and off randomly at different places within the machine. You will be given a response button to hold, and you should press the button whenever you think you have seen a light flash. The best time to blink is right after you have pushed the button. Some lights will be bright and some will be dim; some lights will be too dim to be seen and there will be periods of time when you won't see anything. Don't be alarmed by this -- the machine purposely makes some of the lights too dim as it tries to measure the sensitivity of your eye at various points.

During the examination, you will hear various noises as the light projector moves and the shutter opens and closes. Try to ignore these noises and respond only to the lights -- the machine periodically tests your responses by either not projecting any lights (to see if you are responding to the noises) or by projecting very bright lights (to see if you are paying attention).

This examination can be quite long and tiring, and can take up to 20 minutes per eye. It is most important that you be seated comfortably with your forehead pushed forward into the machine as far as possible. You should feel relaxed with no tension in your shoulders or neck. The fixation light should be clearly in focus. If you are not comfortable or if the light is not in focus, tell the technician immediately. If you wish to rest during the examination simply hold down the response button -- the machine will beep and alert the technician to pause the test.

It is hoped that this information will make visual field testing easier for you. Please do not hesitate to ask the technician or your doctor to explain anything that is not clear to you.

Figure 4-16. A patient information sheet for visual field testing.

response button. This will alert the technician that a rest period is desired and the test can be paused. Other points to emphasize include the information that needs to be communicated back to the operator so that adjustments in the test situation can be made. If the patient does not tell the technician that he or she is uncomfortable or that the inside of the bowl is not in focus, the test will proceed and meaningless results will be obtained. Such patients will certainly not be happy hearing that the test needs to be repeated. All instructions should be reinforced verbally and repeated as often as necessary both before and during the test to make sure that the patient understands and is performing as well as possible. Patients with prior experience with automated perimetry should still read the instructions prior to each test in order to reinforce the above information. There is a learning curve in automated perimetry, and it may take up to four examinations before a patient is fully "seasoned." Written and verbal instructions, repeated as necessary as the test proceeds, may

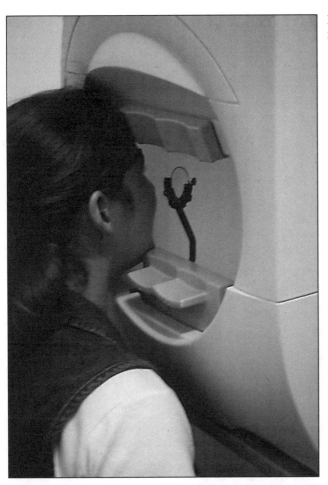

Figure 4-17. A patient improperly positioned in the machine.

help to flatten the learning curve for the patient and make the results more accurate and reliable. Onscreen instructions are also available. Reading such instructions to all patients, and to each patient at every test, serves to standardize the procedures, even with different examiners. A combination of written instructions, reviewed by the patient while the machine is being set up, standardized verbal instructions such as those available in the machine, and additional reinforcement with the opportunity to answer the patient's questions prior to the start of the examination is optimal.

POSITIONING

Once the machine and patient are ready, the patient must be properly positioned. The patient should be seated comfortably on a reasonably soft chair with the neck, shoulders, and arms relaxed. The machine should be at such a height that the patient's forehead is in contact with the head rest when the chin is placed into the chin rest with no tendency to fall back. Figure 4-17 shows a patient improperly positioned in the machine. The positioning in Figure 4-18 is also incorrect, as the table is too low. This patient will become uncomfortable in a short time due to the forced hunching of the shoulders and kinking of the neck. Figure 4-19, although at first glance appears to be alright, shows the effect of the table being too high. The patient has to stretch her neck to reach the head strap. Shortly after beginning the test, her head will fall away from the machine, leaving a large space between her eye and the correcting lens. This can lead to artifactual visual field loss, as discussed later. The patient shown in Figure 4-20 is positioned properly, with the machine set at the proper height.

Once the table height is set and the patient is seated properly, have the patient sit back and place the occluder over the nontested eye, making sure that the eye is completely covered and the elastic strap does not cover the eye being tested. Reposition the patient in the machine and adjust the chin rest height and position

Figure 4-18. Table too low, forcing the patient to bend too far.

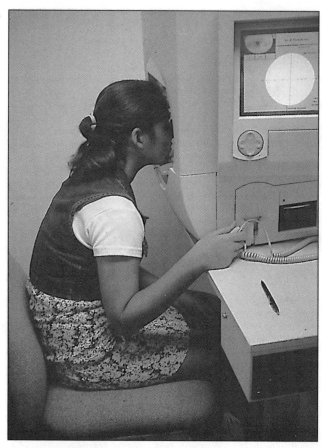

so that the tested eye is centered between the hash marks of the video eye monitor or within the circles of the viewing telescope. The correcting lens is then brought as close as possible to the eye without touching it or the eyelashes. Figure 4-21 shows what can happen if the correcting lens is not properly positioned. The lens holder in this case is too high (or the eye too low), allowing the black casing of the lens holder to block out the inferior portion of the visual field. This may be mistaken for loss due to disease. Other examples of lens malpositioning and correcting lens artifact are given in Chapter 5.

Once everything seems ready, ask the patient if he or she feels comfortable and if the fixation target is in focus. Make any necessary corrections prior to proceeding. Make sure the patient understands what is going to happen and run the demonstration program if necessary. When the patient voices understanding of the procedure, begin the test. Figure 4-22 shows the appearance of the CRT and video eye monitor with the patient and correcting lens properly positioned, ready for the test to begin.

The pupil size may be measured with a millimeter rule directly on the video eye monitor since the magnification is 1:1. For machines equipped with the telescope, the three circles inside correspond to two, four, and six millimeters and pupil size can be estimated by comparing to the circles. Don't forget to enter the pupil size into the patient data screen so that the information will print with the test results. Some models of the 700 series determine pupil size automatically, and the measurement will appear on the printouts.

Administering the Test

The patient should never be left alone during the actual performance of the examination. The technician administering the test can monitor test performance by watching the CRT. The current point being tested will flash on the screen, and the result will appear when the machine is finished with that point. Periodic coaching and encouragement, such as "You're doing fine, Mrs. Jones," or "Just a few more minutes to go," can be

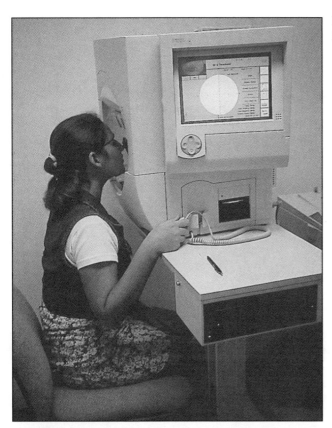

Figure 4-19. Table too high, forcing patient to stretch her neck.

extremely helpful in increasing the patient's level of comfort. The remaining time can be estimated by the number of points that have not been completed. Watch closely for false positive and negative errors, and re-instruct the patient after each error. A running tally of the catch trials is kept in the lower right-hand corner of the screen. The machine beeps with each false response or fixation loss, and the tally can be checked to see which type of error has occurred. False positive responses, false negative responses, and fixation losses are measures of reliability, which are discussed in detail in Chapter 5. For example, if the patient has just made a false positive error (indicating that he or she pushed the response button when no stimulus had been projected), remind him or her to push the button only when a light is seen. Similarly, if a false negative error is made (indicating that the patient failed to push the button when a bright stimulus was flashed in an area that the machine has already determined to have vision), check to make sure that the patient is paying attention, is comfortable, does not want to rest, etc.

The technician must be more than a babysitter during the performance of the test. Even though the machine uses a sophisticated algorithm to monitor fixation, it is important for the operator to carefully monitor the patient's fixation as well during the examination. The patient's eye should remain centered between the hash marks of the video eye monitor or within the center circle of the telescope at all times. It is natural for the patient to look toward where the stimulus was projected, but this should occur after the response button was pushed and should be followed by a rapid shift back to the fixation target. If a lot of random eye movements are observed, remind the patient to try to look steadily at the yellow fixation target. If, despite what appears to be rock steady fixation as determined by patient observation or the Gaze Tracker (models 740 and 750), the machine continues to record fixation losses, it may indicate that the blind spot is incorrectly located or that the blind spot check size is too large. This is discussed in Chapter 5. The technician should pause the test and remap the blind spot, and if the fixation losses persist, change the blind spot check size to a smaller stimulus, such as a I or II. Performing fixation loss catch trials with a stimulus size I does not affect the performance of the visual field test with a size III.

Finally, a test should not be allowed to proceed if the patient does not appear to be responding to the stimuli. If the patient understands the test procedure and has advanced visual field loss, a field full of zeros is

Figure 4-20. Table height set just right for this patient.

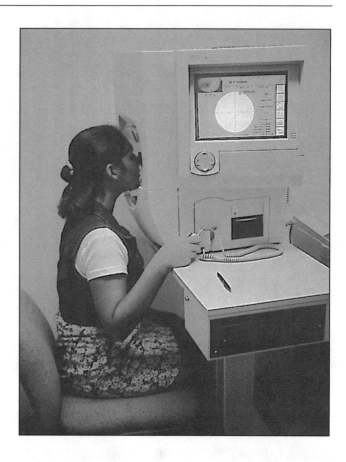

Figure 4-21. The lens holder artifact, resulting from positioning the correcting lens too high relative to the patient's eye.

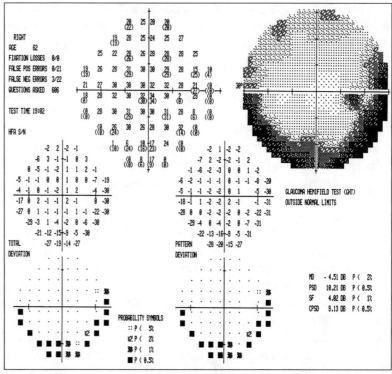

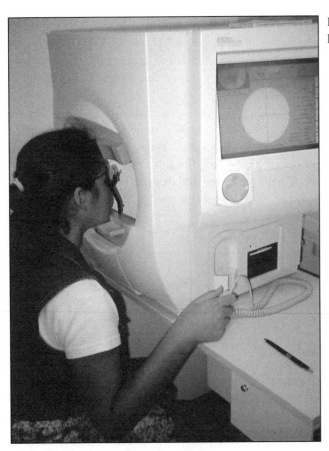

Figure 4-22. The patient and correcting lens properly positioned for the start of the test.

worthless. The test should be stopped and restarted with a larger stimulus, such as size V. Similarly, a patient who proves to be physically incapable of performing a full threshold test should be tried with a simpler test, such as a screen. The decision to deviate from the requested test is that of the operator's and is based on the patient's ability. If in doubt, check with the ordering provider prior to continuing. Any changes from the ordered examination should be fully documented and explained in the medical record and be signed and dated by the examiner.

After the Test

Immediately after the test has concluded, save the results to the disks. Since the Humphrey Field Analyzer 600 series does not automatically default to saving the test results, the operator must push the "save on disk" button. Even though the results of the first eye are saved in memory until the machine is turned off or another patient is tested, saving the results before testing the other eye will help to cut down on lost data. Newer versions of the software have an "auto-save" feature that is selectable from the configuration menu. If this is available, it is highly recommended that it be used. This feature will save the results of the test to both drives immediately upon conclusion of the test. Data saved but later determined to be unnecessary can be deleted, but data not saved can never be recovered.

At the conclusion of a visual field test using one of the HFA II models, two beeps will sound and you will have the option to save the results, to print a hard copy of the test results, or to test the other eye. As with the HFA 600 series, it is a good idea to save the test results before proceeding to test the fellow eye. When saving the results to disk, a prompt will appear on the screen asking for confirmation of the patient's name and date of birth prior to saving the test.

After allowing the patient to rest for as long as necessary, proceed with testing the other eye. Again, do not forget to ensure comfort, centration (and correctness) of the correcting lens, and proper positioning of the patient. Save the results at the conclusion of the test and print out the results according to what the clinician requested. If STATPAC is installed, all patients who have had prior testing should have STATPAC overview and change analysis printouts covering all of their previous examinations and single field analysis of the present examination. Glaucoma patients should have the glaucoma change probability plot printed in lieu of other time series printouts.

Finally, the technician should record comments on the visual field order form or document the performance in the medical record. Items of particular importance are fixation behavior, understanding of the test, cooperation, attitude, and anything else that is felt to be important. The order form with the comments and initials of the technician should be placed in the patient's chart along with the field printouts for review by the provider. Notes written in the record by the technician should be signed and dated. The input provided by the administrator of the test to the clinician is very helpful in interpreting the results and will be discussed further in Chapter 5.

A checklist for visual field technicians is provided in Figure 4-23.

Visual Field Technician Checklist

1. Pull patient's yellow card from the file or create a new one if new patient. Fill in all information.

2. Check visual field order form for appropriate information, including refraction to be used.

3. Set up machine for test using information on the patient data card and the order form. Place corrective lens in holder, using age appropriate add on top of specified distance prescription. If dilated or aphakic use +3.00 add.

4. Position patient -- make sure table height and chin rest are adjusted properly to assure patient comfort. Ask the patient if he/she is comfortable and make appropriate corrections.

5. Measure pupil size on CRT and record on the patient data screen.

6. Enter patient information into machine, including refraction used and pupil size. Make sure birth date and year are correct (do not enter *this* year). Make sure patient's name is entered identically to previous tests.

7. Patient should have read the handout "Visual Field Testing -- Information for Patients." Instruct patient as to nature of test and its performance. Read the instructions to patient from the machine. Make sure the patient understands the procedure and answer any questions before proceeding.

8. Make sure patient understands anticipated length of the test and knows how to rest by holding down the response button.

9. Occlude the untested eye, reposition patient, check position of corrective lens, recheck patient's position, make necessary adjustments, and proceed.

10. Every one or two minutes check the patient's fixation and position in the video eye monitor. Pause and make adjustments as necessary.

11. NEVER LEAVE THE ROOM FOR ANY REASON WHILE A TEST IS BEING PERFORMED. MONITOR THE PATIENT AND THE SCREEN AT ALL TIMES.

12. Re-instruct the patient every time a false positive or false negative response occurs, or if fixation deviation is noted. Offer periodic encouragement and reassurance. Advise when close to finished.

13. SAVE THE RESULTS.

14. Allow brief rest period, and, when patient is ready, proceed with the other eye. Go back to step 3.

15. At conclusion of second eye, print the results according to the order form. Answer the questions at the bottom of the order form and make any comments deemed necessary. Place the printouts and the order form in the patient's chart.

Figure 4-23. A checklist for visual field technicians.

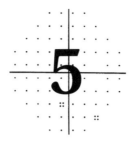

Basic Principles of
Visual Field Interpretation

Introduction

Interpretation of automated fields can be a complex activity when all factors are considered. By using a logical and consistent approach, this task can be made easier. This chapter will discuss such an approach, review reliability measures, present examples of artifact commonly seen in automated fields, provide some guidelines for recognizing true field abnormalities, and discuss the statistical analysis of visual fields.

When "confronted" with a printout from the field analyzer, the following must be considered in order to make a meaningful interpretation:

1. Which test was done?
2. How was the test done (ie, what strategy was used)?
3. What is the reliability of the test?
4. Could any of the defects present represent artifact as opposed to real disease?

Once this information has been ascertained, interpretation may proceed, looking for areas in the field that show true departures from normal. "Normal" is a difficult concept in automated perimetry. On the Humphrey Field Analyzer, "normal" may refer to anticipated values for an individual eye based on test initialization—the anticipated values are those of a hill of vision with the same shape as would be expected in the general population. If using the optional STATPAC software, "normal" refers to the actual average threshold measurements at each point in the grid for a population of the same age as the patient. Some guidelines for determining whether a field or points in a field show "no defect" or are truly abnormal will be presented later in this chapter. Next, try to identify patterns of loss associated with known disease processes, looking for diffuse as well as local depressions indicative of scotomata. Remember to look at the visual fields from both eyes for indications of neurological disease (loss patterns respecting the vertical midline), as well as for asymmetric changes that could be indicative of early glaucomatous damage. Finally, if previous fields have been performed, check for changes over time. Fields may show stability, worsening, or improvement, but bear in mind that these changes may be due not only to disease processes but to test performance factors and variability as well. Clinical correlation follows interpretation; first interpret the field and then correlate the findings with the patient's clinical history and physical findings. Interpretation in this manner serves to eliminate bias in interpretation and allows visual field testing to take its rightful place as a clinical adjunct in the work-up and management of patients.

Figure 5-1. Standard Humphrey Field Analyzer three-in-one printout.

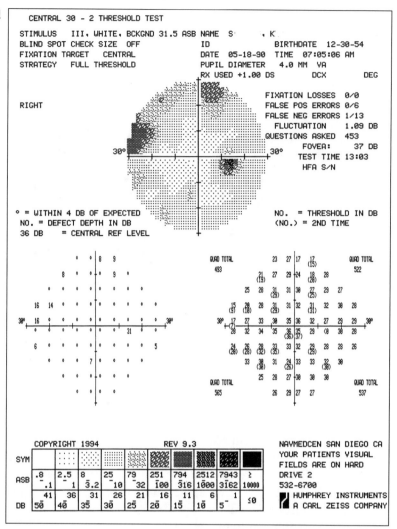

Preliminary Steps in Visual field Interpretation: Identify the Test Performed and How it Was Performed (Strategy)

Figure 5-1 is an example of the standard (non-STATPAC) three-in-one or triple printout from a patient with early glaucomatous visual field loss. The available test grids for both screening and threshold testing and the strategy options have been described in Chapter 2. The name of the test performed is found at the top of the printout from the Humphrey Field Analyzer. It will indicate whether the test was a screening or threshold test as well as what test grid was used (eg, central 30-2 threshold test, full field 120-point screening test, etc). It is important to note this first, since the numbers on the printouts have different meanings depending on whether the test was a suprathreshold screening test or an actual measurement of threshold at each point in the field. Screening and threshold testing are discussed in Chapter 1, printout appearance and symbols for screening tests are discussed in Chapter 2. For some test patterns, the spacing of the test points may look identical when in fact the resolution of the tests differ dramatically. For example, the central 30-2 and central 10-2 on first glance look like the same pattern of points. The resolution of the 30-2 is 6°, while that of the 10-2 is 2°. The easiest way to differentiate between the two is by looking at the name at the top (and the absence of a blind spot on the 10-2). Patient descriptive data is found underneath the test name, followed by the test parameters (stimulus size, blind spot check status, fixation target, correcting lens used, visual acuity, and pupil size) and the strategy used. Verify that all of the information is correct. Knowing the strategy used is particularly important for screening tests, since the symbols used on the printouts have different meanings depending on the strategy. For example, the small black square indicates a point departing from normal by at least six decibels when the threshold-related strategy is used for a screen, but indicates an absolute defect (failure to respond to 10,000 asb [apostilb]) on the three-zone strategy printout. For threshold tests, it is important to recognize if fast-threshold strategy has been used, since this test technique has no way of determining if a visual field has improved. Reliability indices on standard printouts are listed on the right side for right eyes and on the left side for left eyes; they always appear on the left side of the STATPAC printout. The glaucoma hemifield test results are on the right side of the STATPAC printout just below the graytone plot, and the visual field indices are found just below that. An example of a STATPAC single-field analysis and discussion of this software option will be given later in this chapter.

Reliability

Having established which test was performed and how it was performed, next determine if it was reliable. A test that meets the manufacturer's criteria for unreliability may still be a clinically useful test, and an otherwise reliable test may be worthless for establishing a diagnosis or proving that a condition has worsened. The reliability measures available to the eye care professional should be used in conjunction with all available clinical information before a test is discarded. Five measures of reliability can be used: false positive response rate, false negative response rate, fixation losses, fluctuation, and technician comments.

FALSE POSITIVE RESPONSES

During the performance of any visual field test, the Humphrey Filed Analyzer will periodically move the projector and open the shutter without projecting a stimulus. If the patient pushes the response button to this nonprojected stimulus it will be recorded as a false positive response and the machine will beep to alert the technician that a false response has occurred. A running tally of false responses is kept in the lower right-hand corner of the video display. At each occurrence of a false positive response, the technician should make a comment to the patient as a reminder to push the button only when a light is seen. Most patients will have some false positive responses during the test, and up to a 20% rate may be considered acceptable. If the patient's rate exceeds 33%, the printout will indicate so by printing "xx" next to the rate ("xx" next to any of the indices is considered unacceptable by the machine and indicative of unreliability). A high rate of false positives may indicate a patient who is "button-happy." A high rate may also occur when the patient does not understand the test or has a high anxiety level and is concerned with seeing all the lights in order not to be labeled "blind." False positive responses can also occur if the patient learns to respond to machine noise instead of the light. It is easy to get into the rhythm of the whir of the translation motors and the click of the shutter opening, usually followed by a light prompting a push of the response button—whir-click-push, whir-click-push, etc. The cycle may be completed by the button push even if no light was seen, resulting in a false positive response. Later models of the Humphrey Field Analyzer have attempted to limit machine noise by using a "quiet board," but this does not totally eliminate the noises. Some patients still appear to respond to the noise rather than the light. A high false positive rate makes the measured field look better than it really is. In general, a high false positive response rate is the best indication of unreliability, and, unlike the other reliability measures, has no other meaning except that of unreliability.

High false positive responses may affect the field in a number of ways. Sporadic false positive responses scattered over the field may give rise to areas of falsely high sensitivity: the "white scotoma." Figure 5-2 is an example of an unreliable visual field showing 7/16 false positive responses (44%). The graytone printout shows multiple white scotomata, corresponding to areas of abnormally high sensitivity. The circled test points in the figure show threshold values that are impossible (ie, the stimulus intensities would be too dim to be seen even by the most sensitive retina under the best test conditions). Since the patient was pushing the button when he really wasn't seeing the lights, the machine kept making the stimuli dimmer until the patient stopped responding. This field is unreliable and must be repeated if it is to have any clinical usefulness. Figure 5-3 is a more extreme example, showing 90% false positive catch trials. Figure 5-4 is the ultimate in

Figure 5-2. Unreliable visual field due to high false positive responses. Points showing virtually impossible sensitivity are circled.

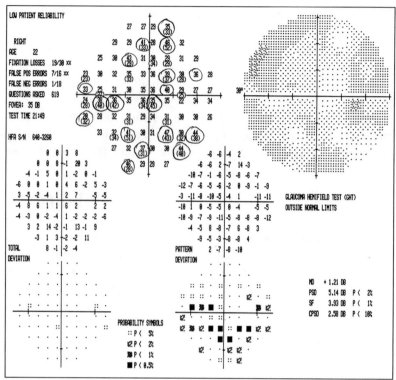

Figure 5-3. An almost white visual field due to 90% false positive responses.

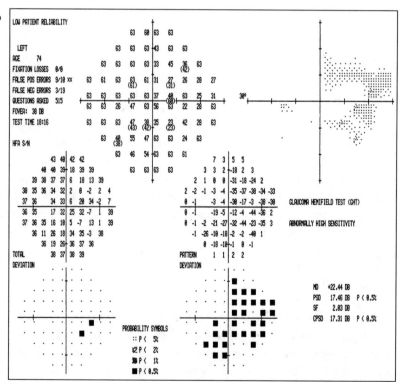

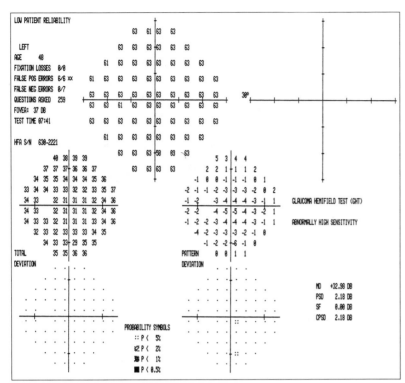

Figure 5-4. Completely white visual field due to 100% false positive responses.

false positive responses—100%! Almost every point in the field shows a value in excess of 60 dB, the dimmest stimuli available on the Humphrey Field Analyzer—values that are undetectable by the human visual system. These patients need careful re-instruction and retesting. The technician should be monitoring for such responses and should never allow an examination to proceed if the patient continues making false responses. It is the job of the technician administering the test to find out what the problem is. Whether it is a matter of comprehension, anxiety, discomfort, inability to focus inside the bowl, or whatever, correct it and then allow the exam to conclude. "Garbage in, garbage out" applies to automated perimetry, and the technician's job is to help keep the garbage to a minimum in order to provide the clinician with meaningful data.

FALSE NEGATIVE RESPONSES

As the test proceeds, the machine identifies areas in which the patient has vision (ie, some points at which threshold measurements were obtainable). During the course of the examination, the machine will come back to a seeing area and project the brightest available stimulus (10,000 asb). Failure to respond to the brightest stimulus in an area previously determined to have some sensitivity is a false negative response. As with false positives, a beep sounds with each occurrence and a tally is kept on the screen. High false negatives may indicate lack of attentiveness, fatigue, or "hypnosis." Some patients may even fall asleep toward the end of a long test. The technician should be alert to this and talk to the patient after each false negative response, pausing the test if necessary to allow rest. In general, a high false negative rate (greater than 20%, although the machine defaults to 33%) makes the field look worse than it really is. However, small (undetectable) shifts in fixation in a patient with marked visual field loss may result in projection of stimuli into a scotoma when it previously was in the seeing field, resulting in a high false negative rate. Fields should not be considered unreliable solely based upon the false negative response rate, particularly if there is a great deal of pathology. The patient in Figure 5-5 has far advanced glaucomatous optic nerve damage. He exhibits 50% false negative responses, which can be attributed to small shifts in fixation. With only very small areas of reasonable sensitivity remaining (circled points), it does not take much movement for a projected stimulus to land in a blind area. This field is otherwise acceptable and is consistent with severe damage. The visual field in Figure 5-6 shows 100% false negative responses and most likely indicates that the patient did not know what to do. Indeed, this test was this patient's first visual field. Figure 5-4 is her second attempt after being instructed to push the button when she thought she saw a light!

Figure 5-5. High false negatives most likely resulting from small shifts in fixation in a severely damaged visual field. Points remaining with relatively good sensitivity are circled—these are most likely the points used for the false negative catch trials.

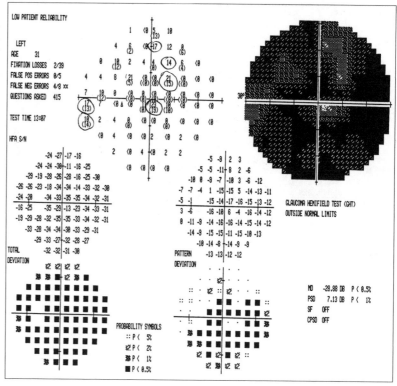

Figure 5-6. One hundred percent false negative responses giving a black field. This is the same patient as Figure 5-4 prior to re-instruction.

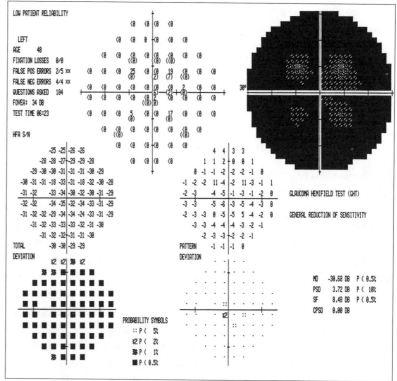

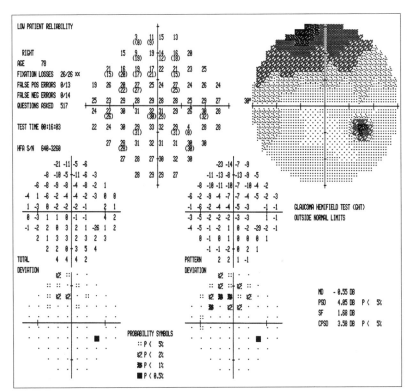

Figure 5-7. One hundred percent fixation losses resulting from proper localization of the blind spot followed by performance of the test while fixating on the lower fixation target instead of the center.

FIXATION LOSSES

The Humphrey Field Analyzer has the capability of monitoring fixation behavior of the patient and determining if fixation losses have occurred. In addition to the gaze tracker (available in the 700 series), discussed in Chapter 2, the Humphrey Field Analyzer may also use the Heijl-Krakau method. At the beginning of each test, the machine will locate the blind spot by serially presenting suprathreshold stimuli around the presumed blind spot until the boundaries are located. A small triangle will appear on the video display and the printout, indicating the location of the blind spot. During the test itself, every 11th stimulus will be projected into the center of the mapped blind spot. A patient response to this stimulus presentation is presumed to have resulted from a shift of fixation. The number of fixation losses and trials is kept as a running tally on the video display during the test with a beep at each occurrence to allow the technician to remind the patient about fixating steadily on the target. Twenty percent fixation loss is considered unreliable. Although a high fixation loss rate may indicate poor fixation behavior and unreliability, fixation deviations should also be monitored by the technician through the telescope or video eye monitor. It is possible in some patients that the blind spot is smaller than the area of the stimulus used to check for fixation losses, thus the projected stimulus would fall on a seeing retina with a resultant false recording of a fixation loss. Incorrect location of the blind spot or a shift in the patient's position after the test has started may give a high fixation loss rate despite actual good fixation behavior. High false positives may also result in a high fixation loss rate, since the patient is inappropriately pushing the button anyway. If the observed fixation behavior is better than the fixation loss rate would indicate, consider decreasing the size of the stimulus used for checking fixation losses (this can be done without changing the stimulus size used for the test itself) or pause the test and remap the blind spot. If you wish to rely on the technician to monitor fixation behavior, you can save approximately 10% of test time by turning off the fixation monitor.

An unusual cause for high fixation losses is shown in Figure 5-7. The blind spot was correctly localized, indicated by the small triangle just below the horizontal meridian 15° temporal to fixation (fixation is at the intersection of the vertical and horizontal axes; each hash mark on the axes is 10°). However, the patient performed the test while fixating on the lower fixation target in the bowl. This served to move his actual blind spot down; this point measured four decibels and then zero decibels and appears as the black spot below the horizontal on the graytone. Since the machine thought the blind spot was in the area indicated by the triangle and the eye was rotated down, each fixation loss catch trial was in actuality projected onto a seeing retina and elicited a response, resulting in the 100% fixation loss rate recorded. Care must be taken in all aspects of test performance to avoid such problems.

TECHNICIAN COMMENTS

Automated perimetry offers the advantage of decreasing the burden placed on the technician in the performance of visual field testing. However, the role of the technician in assuring the quality of the examination is increased since the actual performance of the test is left to the computer, and the technician is removed from this important interactive phase. The technician must assume an active role in the exam, from the initial greeting of the patient through the printout of the examination results. Patients are human beings, not machines, and may require periodic reminders as to what is expected of them during a perimetric examination. Thus, it is imperative that the technician remains in the room with the patient at all times during the test, not only to supply reinstruction when needed as outlined above, but to act as a source of reassurance and comfort as the patient plods through what is often a difficult task. In this role as instructor, the technician becomes a valuable source of information for the person who needs to interpret the results of the examination. Technicians should be encouraged to write, either on the printout or the patient's chart, some comments as to the patient's performance during the test. Comment should include fixation behavior (recorded fixation losses not withstanding and mandatory if the fixation monitor is turned off), ability to understand the test procedures, ability to perform the test, fatigue and when it occurred (which eye, tired before the beginning of the examination, etc), cooperation, general attitude, any comments the patient may have made, etc. These comments can be invaluable in interpreting the test results and understanding the other reliability measures as recorded by the machine. It may be useful to list some of this desired information directly on the visual field ordering form as "yes/no" questions, which the technician can quickly answer at the conclusion of the examination. This can then be reviewed along with the visual field printout. The visual field order form is discussed in Chapter 4 under test ordering, and the technician questionnaire appears at the bottom of the form.

FLUCTUATION

Variability in responses is inherent to threshold perimetric testing. The definition of threshold (that value of light intensity which has a 50% probability of being seen), combined with the ever present "human" factors, give rise to this variability, or fluctuation, in measured thresholds. However, variability of response should, under normal circumstances, have a limit. In general, during one test session, a patient's measured threshold on repeat measurements at the same point should be within one to two decibels of each other. Wider spread than this (greater than 2.5 dB and certainly greater than three decibels) may have implications either on reliability or pathology. Fluctuation exists in two different forms: the variability in threshold measurements observed within one test session is referred to as short-term fluctuation, and the variability between threshold measures at the same point found between test sessions (regardless of the interval between those sessions) is known as long-term fluctuation. Short-term fluctuation is considered a reliability measure or indication of instability in the visual field, and long-term fluctuation is considered to determine the change in the field over time. Short-term fluctuation is measured by double-determining threshold at a fixed number of points in the test grid (usually 10), calculating the standard deviation between those measurements, and averaging it over the entire field. The formula for calculating short-term fluctuation and how location of the test points is taken into consideration is discussed along with the visual field indices in the STATPAC section later in this chapter. Test points that have been double-determined will have two numbers appearing at the point location, with the first value on top and the repeat value underneath in parenthesis. It appears on the printout as a fluctuation value. At the present time, the Humphrey Field Analyzer does not offer a numerical measurement of long-term fluctuation.

Patients who truly do not understand the test procedures may show wide variability in their responses. They may therefore be considered unreliable and their results discounted. If this is the case, it should be reflected in the other reliability measures (false positives, false negatives, fixation losses, and technician com-

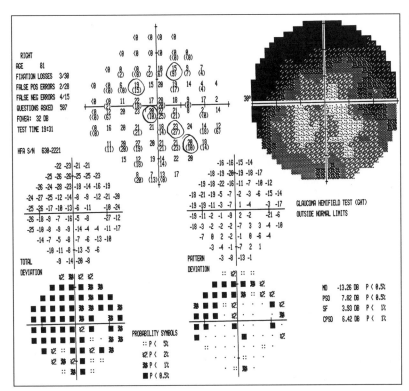

Figure 5-8. High short-term fluctuation in an otherwise reliable visual field. Points of the fluctuation test showing large spread in repeated measures are circled.

ments). However, consider the case of the otherwise reliable patient who shows high fluctuation. It has been shown that fluctuation increases as retinal sensitivity decreases (a light bulb that flickers as it wears out will sometimes be bright and sometimes be dim). Thus, in an otherwise reliable patient, it is imperative to scan the field and look for the points showing high spread (Figure 5-8). Usually, these points will be located within scotomata or at the borders of a scotoma (Figure 5-9). If no scotoma is present, the areas of high fluctuation (in an otherwise reliable field not showing any other defects) are likely to become depressed in the future. Increasing fluctuation may be predictive of impending visual field loss and may be the earliest visual field defect in glaucoma. Like the flickering light bulb, increased fluctuation may mean that something needs to be done before the patient is left in the dark. An example of significant short-term fluctuation is given in Chapter 6, Figure 6-3, and is also discussed later in this chapter with the visual field indices in the section on *Statistical Analysis of Visual Fields*. This patient has glaucoma, some cataract, and age-related macular degeneration with moderate visual field loss. The field shows diffuse depression as well as focal superior loss. The points showing wide spread in repeated threshold determinations are circled. Note that the points showing the most fluctuation are within or at the borders of scotomata. The inferior central point showing the values of 20 dB and 10 dB corresponds to a small pigment epithelial detachment. The field is otherwise reliable, and the increased fluctuation is attributable to loss of sensitivity from disease. Note also the points that have lost all detectable sensitivity (< 0 dB, indicating failure to respond to the brightest available stimulus) do not exhibit any fluctuation ("dead is dead").

Artifact in Automated Perimetry

Not all defects seen on a perimetric test are due to disease requiring treatment. The identification of visual field defects due to disease requires that defects from other causes be excluded. Once again, human factors, both on the part of the patient as well as the examiner, influence the performance and results of the test and may give rise to depressions that may be misinterpreted as being due to disease. Artifact in visual field testing may be defined as apparent visual field loss that is not due to any malfunction of the visual system. One of the hallmarks of artifact in the visual field is its lack of correlation to known disease processes.

Figure 5-9. Another example of increased short-term fluctuation in a patient with glaucoma and a well-defined superior nerve fiber bundle defect. The high value (4.52) arises from the two circled points, both within or at the border of the scotoma.

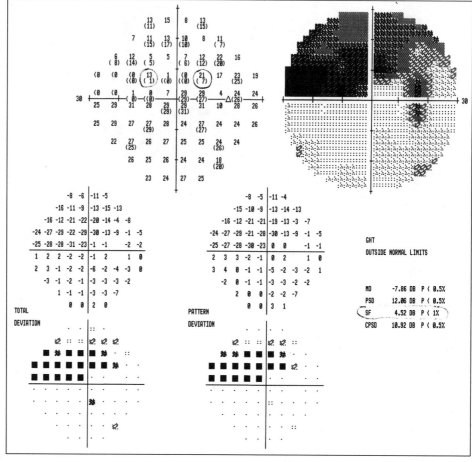

The following are situations that commonly give rise to artifactual visual field loss.

LID AND BROW ARTIFACT

The anatomy of the patient's face and orbit may, on occasion, give rise to visual field defects frequently identified as due to glaucoma. Patients with prominent superior orbital ridges will often manifest superior visual field depressions that may appear to be a superior arcuate scotoma. This type of defect can be properly identified by its lack of connection to the horizontal midline and blind spot, as well as by correlation with the appearance of the patient. Ptotic upper eyelids may give rise to similarly appearing defects. When any doubt exists as to the cause of such defects, it might be prudent to repeat the examination with the lid taped up or with the patient's head tilted back from the headrest in order to roll the eye down.

The patient shown in Figure 5-10 underwent testing twice in the right eye on the same day for reasons that are not entirely clear. The first visual field, performed at 8:30 am, shows basically no defect. The repeat examination at 9:30 am shows a dense superior defect that does not connect to the blind spot. The patient was fatigued and had considerable lid droop when the second examination was performed. Contrast this figure with Figure 5-11, which shows a superior arcuate defect that does connect to the blind spot. Another clue to the nerve fiber bundle origin of this defect is the relatively good sensitivity peripheral to the defect, at least nasally.

CORRECTING LENS ARTIFACT

Make a circle with the thumb and forefinger of your right hand. Close your left eye and look through the circle with your right eye with your hand held against your orbit. Now slowly move your hand away from your eye to a distance of about one to 1.5 inches. As you do this, you will note that a portion of your visual

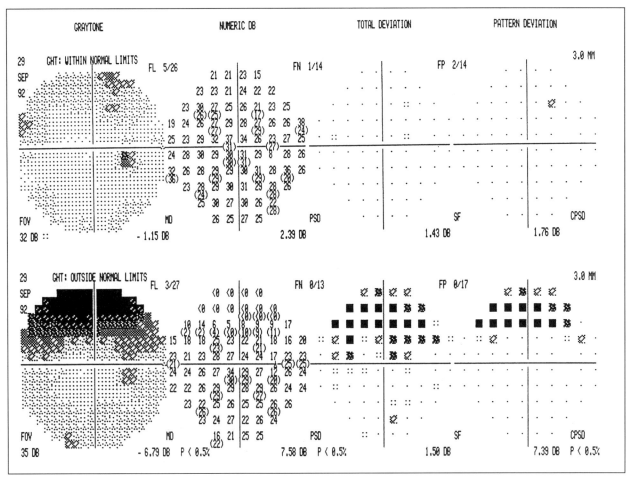

Figure 5-10. A superior defect due to a ptotic upper eyelid found on repeat examination of the same eye within one hour of a normal examination. The droop was most likely due to fatigue.

field is blocked out by the circle made by your fingers. You have just reproduced the ring scotoma that may be seen when the correcting lens used for the visual field test is too far from the patient's eye. The edge of the lens or the lens holder is responsible for the defect. Similarly, if the patient is positioned so that the lens holder is too high relative to the eye, an inferior visual field defect that respects the horizontal midline may be created, which resembles glaucomatous field loss. This defect may be distinguished by its characteristic shape (corresponding to the shape of the lens holder), its lack of connection to the blind spot, and its disappearance upon proper lens positioning. These lens artifacts are more common in patients requiring significant hyperopic correction and are reminiscent of the ring scotoma experienced by patients wearing aphakic spectacles in the days prior to intraocular lenses. Figure 4-21 is the classic rim artifact corresponding precisely to the shape of the correcting lens holder. Figure 5-12 shows the characteristic appearance of another lens rim defect. This field is from a patient with hyperopic correction and a superior ring defect, worse on the temporal side. The defect does not connect to the blind spot. There is no significant loss attributable to disease in this field. Figure 5-13 is a perfect ring, Figure 5-14 is another ring with the lens decentered inferiorly. The patient in Figure 5-15 sought a second opinion after being started on glaucoma medications based upon the illustrated visual field. Her optic nerve was completely normal, and her intraocular pressure following cessation of therapy was 12 mm Hg. Her visual field performed with the lens in the correct position is shown in Figure 5-16.

These defects are avoidable with proper positioning of the patient in the machine and correct placement of the lens and lens holder, as discussed in Chapter 4. Monitoring throughout the examination is essential, for if the patient's head drifts away from the headrest, the lens will be too far from the eye and these defects will appear. Proper positioning at the start of the test does not necessarily guarantee that the patient will

Figure 5-11. A real (nonartifactual) superior defect due to glaucoma. Note the connection of the defect to the blind spot and a few peripheral points showing better sensitivity than the more central areas.

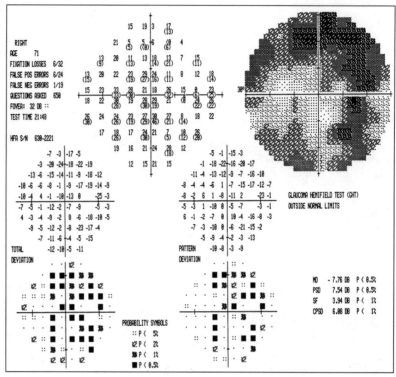

Figure 5-12. A small ring defect.

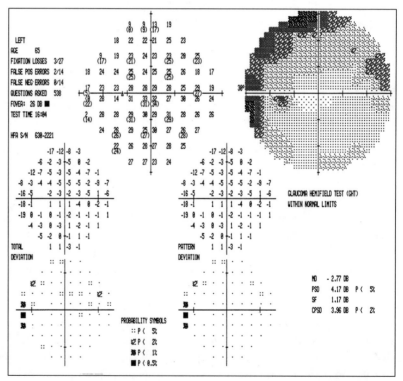

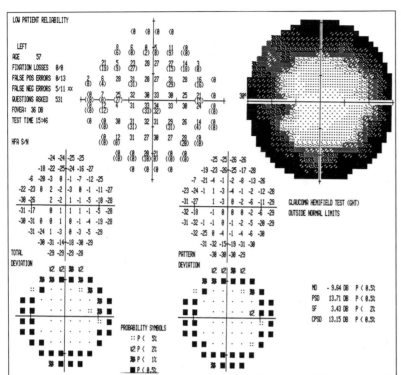

Figure 5-13. A "full-blown" correcting lens defect.

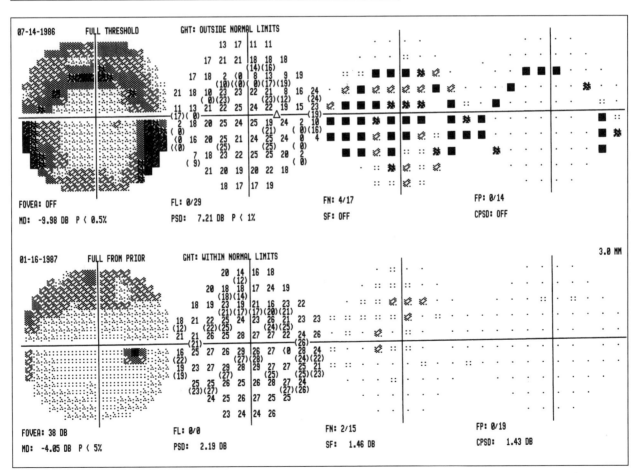

Figure 5-14. Another example of a ring-like scotoma arising due to inferior displacement of the correcting lens (top). The bottom shows the repeat visual field 6 months later with proper placement of the correcting lens.

Figure 5-15. Marked decentration of the lens caused this defect. The patient was started on glaucoma treatment as a result of this visual field.

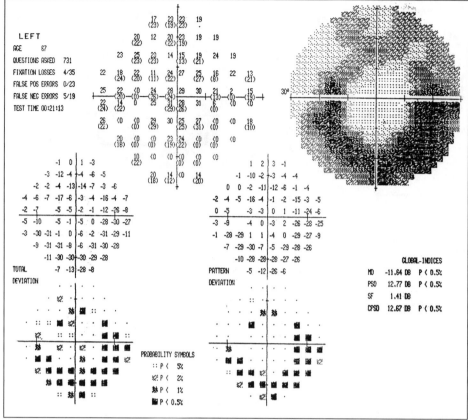

remain in place for the entire examination. The technician should periodically check the patient's head position during the examination and make any necessary adjustments. Repeating an examination when any doubt exists as to the origin of defects cannot be over emphasized.

PUPIL EFFECTS

Constricted pupils are thought to give rise to diffuse visual field depression. Strictly speaking, this is real visual field loss and not artifact, but it should go away if the field is repeated with the pupil dilated. There appears to be a critical size at which pupil size becomes important. In a study involving normal subjects, constriction of the pupil from six to 2.5 mm resulted in uniform (with regard to eccentricity) diffuse depression of the visual field of at most 2.5 dB, which would not be considered clinically significant. Pupils of less than two millimeters are more likely to exert a significant effect on the overall level of the visual field, particularly if a media opacity is present in the visual axis. It is recommended that pupils of less than two millimeters be dilated (if safe to do so). Remember to check the distance refraction after dilation and test with the full add (+3.00) for the test distance, regardless of the patient's age, since a dilated patient has minimal accommodative ability.

Figure 5-17 shows the effect of dilating the pupil in a patient taking pilocarpine. The top examination, performed with the pupil constricted to 1 mm due to pilocarpine, shows mild diffuse depression and a mean deviation of -3.19 dB. The follow-up examination, performed with appropriate refraction following pupillary dilation, shows no defect and a mean deviation of +0.89 dB, an improvement in mean sensitivity of more than four decibels from dilating the pupil. Of course, when dilating the pupils of glaucoma patients, make sure that they do not have occludable angles and make sure to check the intraocular pressure following dilation. Some patients, even with open angles, can have significant increases in intraocular pressure following dilation.

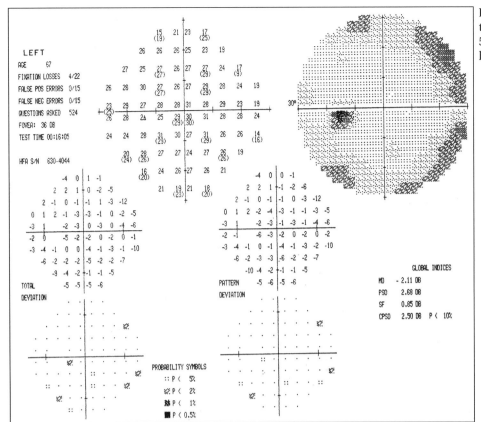

Figure 5-16. Visual field of the patient shown in Figure 5-15 performed with the lens in proper position.

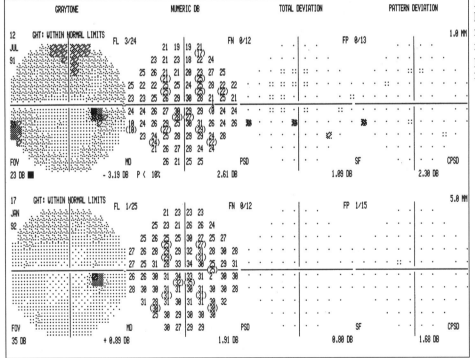

Figure 5-17. Effect of pupillary dilation on the visual field. Note a decrease in mean deviation when the pupil is dilated from one to five millimeters.

Figure 5-18. Diffuse depression resulting from use of the wrong correcting lens.

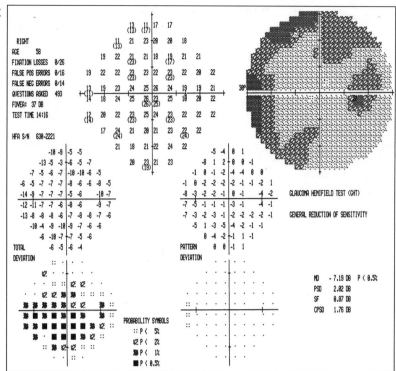

REFRACTIVE ERROR

Errors from lens positioning have been discussed. Artifact also arises from incorrect lens power. The patient must be optically corrected for the test distance in order to properly perceive the projected stimuli. If the targets are not in focus, they will need to be brighter (or larger) in order to be recognized and elicit a response. Thus, incorrect refractive error and/or incorrect calculation of the required add will result in apparent visual field depression. A patient tested without the proper add is shown in Figure 4-15. Figure 5-18 is an example of a patient whose distance refractive error was close to plano. The visual field performed on Sept. 9, 1991 with a +4.75 lens shows diffuse depression with a mean deviation of -7.19 dB. The repeat examination, Figure 5-19, performed the following day with the correct lens (+2.00 0.50 x 180) shows only mild nasal loss and a mean deviation of -0.77 dB. An accurate distance refraction shortly before the examination, or at least assuring that the visual acuity has not changed from the last visit to the day of the visual field examination, combined with selection of the appropriate add as recommended by the manufacturer, is essential to avoid these artifactual defects.

Mistakes in selecting the correcting lens may lead to marked diffuse depression. The patient whose visual fields are presented in Figure 5-20 returned for his visual field examination as scheduled. The field had been ordered six months previously using our ordering form (see Figure 4-12). The specified refractive error was approximately -6.00 in each eye, and the patient was appropriately tested with -3.00 OU. What anyone failed to recognize until after the test was that in the time since the examination was ordered, the patient underwent refractive surgery (LASIK) in each eye and was now plano OU! He therefore should have been tested with +3.00 OU, resulting in a six-diopter error and diffuse depression. Figure 5-21 is a series of examinations from a patient demonstrating a marked overall worsening from April 1992 to October 1993. The examination on October 26, 1993 was performed with a minus lens of the same magnitude as the plus lens that should have been used. Repeat examination two days later shows that the field has not changed from baseline.

It may be useful to measure foveal threshold at the very beginning of the test. If the patient is not properly focused on the interior of the bowl, the foveal sensitivity may be reduced along with the remainder of the field. If it is known that the patient has good visual acuity, a significant reduction in foveal threshold

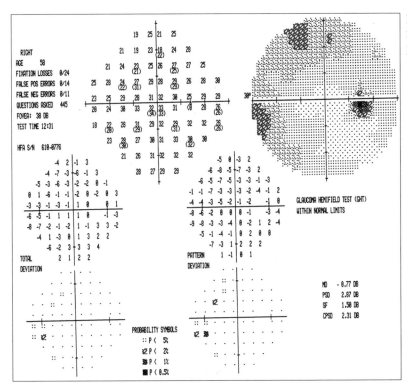

Figure 5-19. Improvement in the visual field when the proper lens is used (same patient as Figure 5-18).

should alert the technician that perhaps the optical correction is not right. Finally, patients should be encouraged to alert the technician if the bowl is not in focus so that the appropriate adjustments can be made. Advising the patient to tell the technician about blurring inside the bowl should be part of the pretest instructions. The patient in Figures 5-18 and 5-19 only shows a one-decibel decrease in foveal threshold on the test with the incorrect lens. However, the patient in Figure 5-21 shows a marked decrease in foveal threshold to 22 dB, which came back up to 37 dB when the correct lens was used.

GRAYTONE CONSTRUCTION ARTIFACT

The Humphrey Field Analyzer graytone printout is a graphic representation of the measured threshold values, designed so that areas of lower retinal sensitivity appear darker, with absolute defects (failure to respond to 10,000 asb stimuli) appearing black. The range of available stimulus intensities from 0 (brightest) to 63 (dimmest) dB is divided into 10 groups, each assigned a symbol of increasing darkness corresponding to decreasing sensitivity. The change in contrast from one group symbol to the next is fairly uniform and should allow easy recognition of areas of depression within areas of greater sensitivity. However, the observer's eye may be fooled by the symbol for the 16 to 20 dB range into thinking that a scotoma exists when it appears next to that of the 21 to 25 dB range when indeed there is no scotoma. Misinterpretation occurs because the contrast between these two symbols is fairly large, with the 16 to 20 dB symbol appearing much darker next to the lighter symbol for 21 to 25 dB. If two adjacent field points have threshold measurements of 21 and 20 dB respectively, the observer may be fooled by the symbols and label the 20 dB point as a scotoma. This is illustrated by the apparent superior arcuate defect shown in Figure 5-22. The graytone symbols are shown at the bottom of the figure (they appear on every Humphrey printout). The symbols for the ranges of 21 to 25 dB and 16 to 20 dB have been highlighted. Note how much darker the 16 to 20 dB symbol appears. This field demonstrates early superior paracentral loss, not nearly as extensive as the graytone would suggest. There is mild diffuse depression in this field, which brings all of the thresholds down into the ranges requiring these symbols. However, the actual focal loss is minimal. This artifact of graytone construction emphasizes the need to look at the value table, rather than the graytone printout, in determining field defects. Statistical analysis, as discussed below, is useful in sorting out true loss from this type of artifact, particularly after the field has been "corrected" for diffuse effects.

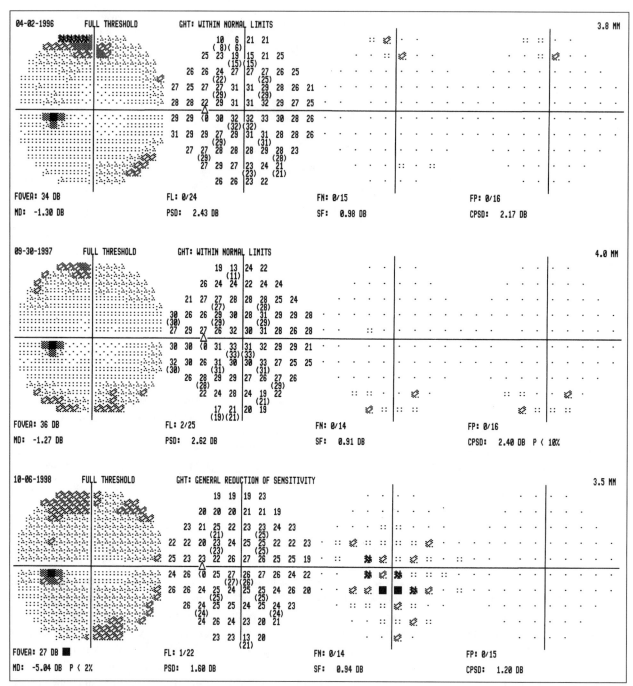

Figure 5-20, left eye. Series of visual fields from both eyes of a glaucoma suspect. This test was ordered four months before the actual date of the exam using the ordering form shown in Chapter 4. The patient's refractive error (approximately -5.00 OU) was entered on the form and the appropriate lens (approximately -2.00 OU) was used by the technician when the October 1998 exam was performed. However, in the time between when the exam was ordered and when it was performed, the patient had LASIK performed on each eye (he didn't tell the technician) and was now emmetropic OU, therefore he should have been tested with a +3.00 OU. The 5 diopter error caused the diffuse depression seen in each eye compared to the previous two exams.

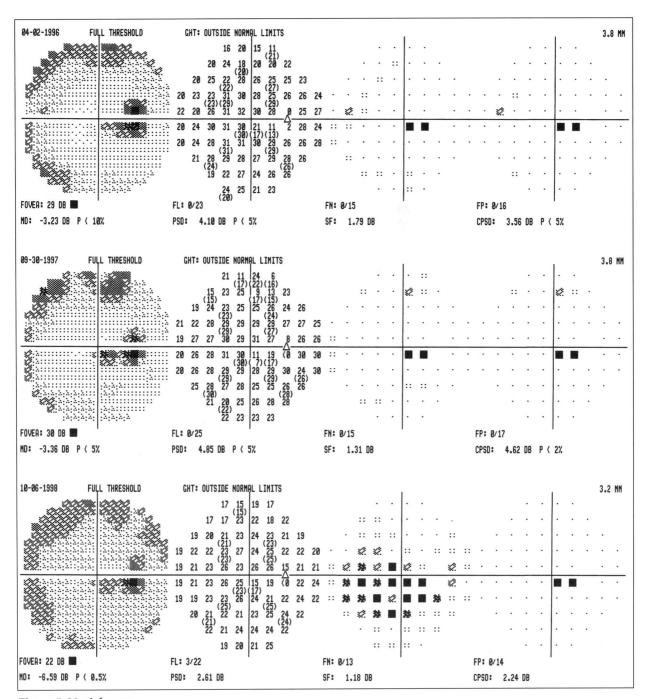

Figure 5-20, right eye.

Figure 5-21. A series of examinations showing apparent worsening attributed to an incorrect lens. Use of the correct lens shows no change from baseline.

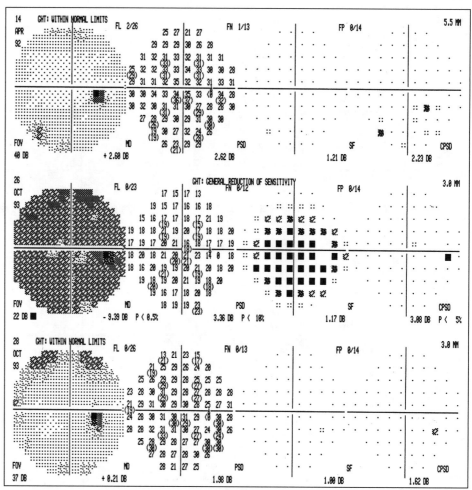

Another example is shown in Figure 5-23. This patient has diffuse depression, but appears on the gray-tone to have an altitudinal defect. When the field is statistically corrected for the diffuse loss, there is only very mild loss present in the superior hemifield compared to the inferior.

"True" Field Abnormalities

True visual field defects, as opposed to artifact, are those that are due to dysfunction of the visual system, either in the eye, optic pathways, or brain. Defects fall into one of two categories: local defects (scotomata) and diffuse defects (overall depression of the visual field). Examples of how automated perimetry displays the various types of local defects that occur in glaucoma, retinal disease, neurological disease, and other ocular conditions will be presented in subsequent chapters.

Diffuse depression of the visual field occurs when the overall height of the field is lowered and all the points show a reduction in sensitivity. This may occur alone or in conjunction with local defects (scotomata). Diffuse depression can be recognized by a lower than expected value for the central reference level (non-STATPAC printouts), an overall "darkening" of the graytone printout, or an increase in the mean deviation on the STATPAC printout. (A single, large, deep or absolute defect may also give rise to a large mean deviation but the other areas in the field will be relatively normal.) Diffuse depression may be seen with media opacities (particularly cataract), pupil effects as discussed above, incorrect refraction, or diffuse optic neuropathy from a variety of causes, glaucoma included. Figure 5-24 is a series of visual fields from the same eye before and after cataract extraction, demonstrating increasing diffuse depression followed by improvement after removal of the cataract in 1989.

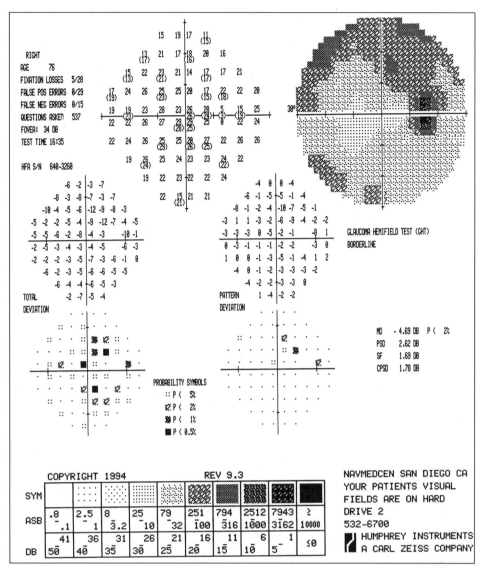

Figure 5-22. The artifact of graytone construction, causing the appearance of more severe visual field loss than is really present.

As previously stated, patient responses and results on automated perimetry are subject to variability and fluctuation. When faced with an apparent defect in the visual field, the question arises how to know that the defect is not the result of this variability. As a rough guideline, a defect depth greater than 2.5 times the short-term fluctuation has a high probability of being a real defect. Remember, this does not necessarily mean that the defect is from disease: it still could be artifact. Clinical correlation and explanation are still required.

The default value for labeling a point as being significantly depressed varies with the program being used and the software installed. On a screening test, for example, a point would have to be more than 6 dB depressed from expected normal to register as a defect. For threshold tests, 4 dB from expected normal is allowed before the defect depth printout will show a point to be defective. On the STATPAC printouts, any departure from normal is shown along with a symbol to indicate the percentage of the reference population expected to show such a defect. In order to avoid overestimating the significance of defects, it is recommended that any single point with a defect depth greater than 10 dB be considered significant, especially if it is found in a point surrounded by "normal" areas. Similarly, clusters of two or more contiguous points showing defect depths of six or more decibels should be considered abnormal. Finally, any defect that persists on repeated testing in a reliable patient has a high probability of being a real defect when compared to "normal." Remember that concepts of normal are with regard to a reference population (either in terms of shape of the hill of vision or actual point-by-point sensitivity) and any individual eye may show a "normal"

Figure 5-23. Another example of the gray-tone construction artifact. This field shows diffuse loss with an apparent altitudinal defect. In reality, only very mild superior loss is present.

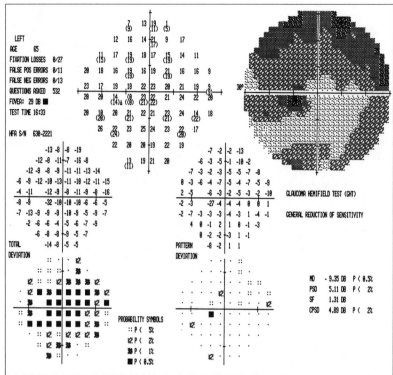

hill of vision that differs from the average. The importance of clinical correlation and explanation for any defect in the field cannot be overemphasized.

Statistical Analysis of Visual Fields

Material in this section is adapted from Choplin N. Technical advances in automated perimetry: statistical analysis of visual fields. *Ophthalmic Practice.* 1992; 10(6):276-283.

GENERAL CONCEPTS OF STATISTICS AS APPLIED TO AUTOMATED PERIMETRY

A statistic is an estimate of the (true) value of a parameter within a population. As such, statistics apply to populations, not individuals, and are derived by sampling the population being studied. Any parameter of a population may be described in terms of a mean (average) value, spread of the measurements around that mean (variance or standard deviation), and a range of normal values. For a normally distributed parameter, values lying outside of the mean value ± two standard deviations are generally considered to be abnormal; the normal range thus encompasses 95% of the measured values. Extreme high and low values would each be expected to occur in less than 2.5% of the population. For example, intraocular pressure in a hypothetical (disease-free) population is normally distributed and determined in a sample of 1000 individuals from that population to have a mean of 16 ± 2.5 mm Hg. Ninety-seven and a half percent of the measurements would be expected to be less than 21 mm Hg. When another individual from that population is found to have an intraocular pressure of 23 mm Hg, he would be considered to be "abnormal" because his measurement lies outside of the normal range. What is important about the observation regarding this individual is that even though the pressure reading is "abnormal," it has little significance in terms of the presence or absence of any disease in this individual. Other factors need to be evaluated to make this determination; thus, the presence of statistical abnormality for an individual compared to the population he comes from must be interpreted in light of the clinical situation.

The parameter of interest in automated perimetry is the threshold at each point in the test grid. When drawing the map of the island of vision for a patient with or suspected of having a disease, the question to

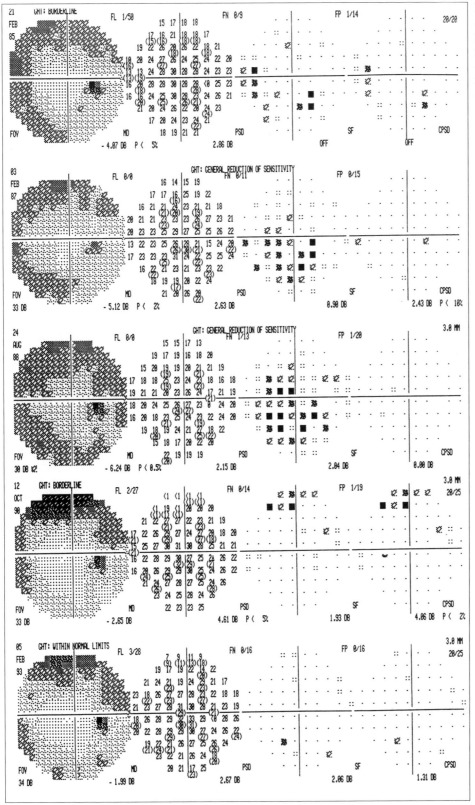

Figure 5-24. Overview analysis of a series of visual fields demonstrating diffuse depression from the development of a cataract, followed by improvement after cataract surgery.

be answered is whether or not the drawn map is "normal." There must therefore be "normal" threshold values derived from disease-free individuals from the same population as the patient at risk. These values can then be used to define the "normal' height and shape of the island of vision for the population. Normal threshold values are derived from measurements (usually repeated) of many individuals from the "normal" population. Each point in the visual field can be assigned an expected normal threshold value based upon the age of the patient (values not directly measured are obtained through linear regression analysis). Although the expected normal value for threshold at each test point in the reference population is not normally distributed (it is negatively skewed), it has a mean, a variance (and standard deviation), and a range of normal. The measured threshold values of the patient can then be compared to the expected population normals, and patient values for each point that lies outside of the range containing 95% of the population measured values can be considered "abnormal." The height and shape of the measured field can also be compared to that of the reference population for abnormality. It must be emphasized, again, that measured threshold values that lie outside of what is statistically normal (ie, "abnormal" may have no clinical significance; interpretation of deviations from normal cannot be made without clinical correlation).

STATISTICAL ANALYSIS FOR THE HUMPHREY FIELD ANALYZER—STATPAC

In the mid-1980s, Allergan-Humphrey introduced an optional statistical analysis package for the Humphrey Field Analyzer called STATPAC, with additions and modifications made available in 1989 as another option called STATPAC 2. These packages allow for the analysis of single visual fields with respect to a normal reference population, as well as for the analysis of a series of tests for changes over time. The package resides within the EPROMs that contain the operating software for the field analyzer and no external computer is required. Adding STATPAC to an existing field analyzer or upgrading from STATPAC to STATPAC 2 is merely a matter of changing the four EPROMs located on the motherboard behind the door on the back panel, which is provided for this purpose. The STATPAC programs are analytical only and in no way change the way in which the testing procedures are carried out; only the output format and data analysis are changed by this software. Analysis of visual fields with STATPAC allows the patient to be compared with a model of the visual field that measures how frequently the threshold result found at a given location in the patient's field occurs in the normal population. The package was developed by Anders Heijl and coworkers, utilizing 487 tests deemed reliable from 239 normal individuals from four different test centers. Through statistical analysis of the data obtained from these 487 fields, "normal" threshold values, more or less corresponding to the mean of the measurements, were derived for each point available in the test contained in the central 30°. In addition, the variance, or spread of measurements around the mean, was determined around each of the mean thresholds for each of the available points, and the data was extrapolated to allow for comparing each patient to a normal of the same age. It is thus known how frequently a particular threshold value could be expected to occur at each of the test points. For a specific patient value, the difference from the mean value in the normal reference population can be determined, as well as what percent of the time such a value would be expected to occur in the normal reference population. A low value, for example, showing a large difference from expected normal, expected to occur in the normal population less than 0.5% of the time, has a very high probability of being "abnormal."

STATPAC is designed for, and can only be used with, central threshold tests that include the 24-1, 24-2, 30-1, and 30-2, utilizing stimulus size III and a white test object. It may not be used on averaged or merged fields. It can be used with previously performed tests that have been stored on floppy disks or the hard drive, as well as later ones, since the analytical package does not change the way the test is performed. Although the package can also be applied to tests performed with the "full from prior data" threshold strategy, it is not meant to be used with such tests and also cannot be used with the fast-threshold strategy. Because STATPAC makes calculations and displays with reference to a database of "normals" of the same age as the patient, it is essential that the patient's birth date be correctly entered.

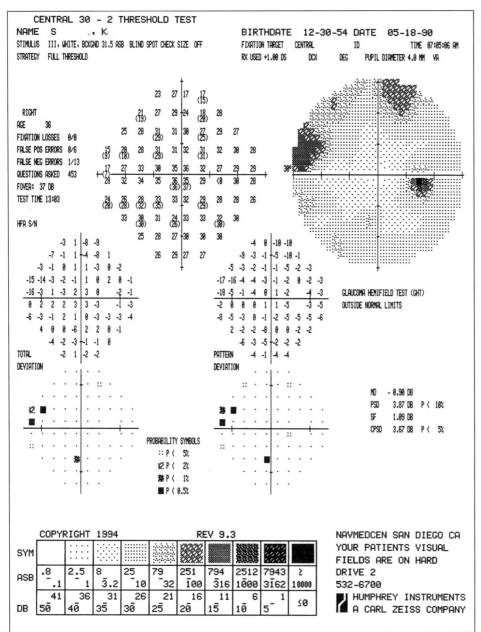

Figure 5-25. Example of a STATPAC single field analysis.

Analysis of a Single Visual Field

Figure 5-25 is an example of a STATPAC single-field analysis. Patient-identifying data and the test performed appear at the top of the page as before. The top grids are the usual patient-measured threshold values (expressed in decibels) and graytone formats, which are no different than those found on the standard Humphrey triple printout. The four bottom grids are the new analyses provided by STATPAC. Three types of analyses are provided for single fields: numerical deviation maps, probability maps, and global indices. STATPAC 2 adds a fourth: the glaucoma hemifield test.

The upper left grid displays the algebraic difference between the measured threshold values and the expected normal value for the patient's age for each test point, labeled "total deviation." A symbol is assigned to each deviation value, indicating the probability of finding such a deviation in the reference population. The darker the symbol, the greater the probability of abnormality (ie, that threshold value is less commonly seen among normal subjects).

Visual field loss, expressed in static perimetry as depressions of sensitivity, occur in two ways: diffuse

Figure 5-26. Unmasking of focal defects in the pattern deviation plot as STATPAC corrects the total deviation plot for diffuse acting effects.

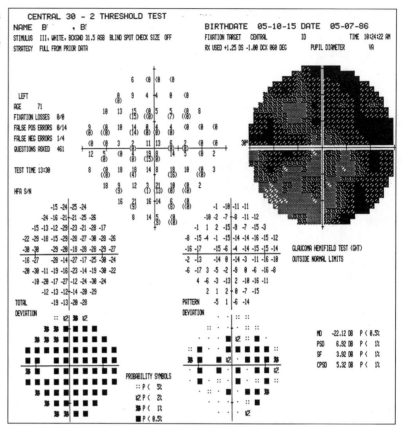

(affecting the entire field, as might occur due to media opacities, incorrect refraction, or small pupils) and local (scotomata). Diffuse loss, in which all of the measured thresholds are below normal (or possibly above normal), can mask focal loss. STATPAC corrects the total deviation plot for diffuse loss, raising or lowering the overall height of the island of vision toward the mean for the reference population and displays the results as the "pattern deviation" plot, printed on the right side of the page. Probability plots are displayed below the plot. This process eliminates or diminishes general changes in height of the measured field while focal loss remains clearly visible or enhanced.

Figure 5-26 is an example of a patient with a dense cataract and advanced glaucomatous damage. The adjustment from total deviation to pattern deviation reveals the nature of the focal loss, which is extensive in this case. Approximately 14 dB has been "added back" to the depressions noted on the total deviation plot. This "adjustment" is based on the distribution of the deviations noted in the total deviation plot. The "correcting factor" applied to generate the pattern deviation plot is that value of deviation from the total deviation plot that lies at the 92nd percentile, with some consideration given for the location of each point as it is "corrected." The four values given on the extreme right of the printout are the "global indices" (labeled MD, PSD, SF, and CPSD) These indices represent reductions in field data to single numbers and serve to summarize the field data. Probability (P) values are given for values outside of the normal range, indicating what percentage of the reference population may be expected to show the same or larger value. The formulas for calculating the indices can be found in Figure 5-27. It is important to note that the calculation of each index takes into consideration the location of each test point; since the normal database contains the variance of each point around its mean value, these calculation methods allow deviations in the center of the field to be given more significance than equivalent deviations in the periphery where the variance is greater.

The indices are:

Mean deviation (MD): in general, a measure of the overall height of the island of vision with regard to the reference population (ie, an estimate of the uniform part of the deviation from normal). It is actually a measure of the average deviation of the island of vision with regard to the reference population (ie, an estimate of the total deviation from normal, localized, as well as diffuse). A negative number implies that the

$$MD = \left(\frac{1}{n} \sum_{i=1}^{n} \frac{(x_i - N_i)}{s_{1_i}^2} \right) \bigg/ \left(\frac{1}{n} \sum_{i=1}^{n} \frac{1}{s_{1_i}^2} \right)$$

where x_i is the measured threshold at point i, N_i is the normal reference threshold at point i, s_{1i}^2 is the variance of normal field measurements at point i, and n denotes the number of test points, excluding the blind spot.

$$PSD = \sqrt{ \left(\frac{1}{n} \sum_{i=1}^{n} s_{1_i}^2 \right) * \left(\frac{1}{n-1} \sum_{i=1}^{n} \frac{(x_i - N_i - MD)^2}{s_{1_i}^2} \right) }$$

where x_i is the measured threshold at point i, N_i is the normal reference threshold at point i, s_{1i}^2 is the variance of normal field measurements at point i, n denotes the number of test points, excluding the blind spot, and MD is the mean deviation.

$$SF = \sqrt{ \left(\frac{1}{10} \sum_{j=1}^{10} s_{2_j}^2 \right) * \left(\frac{1}{10} \sum_{j=1}^{10} \frac{(x_{j_1} - x_{j_2})^2}{2 * s_{2_j}^2} \right) }$$

where x_{j1} is the first threshold measurement at each of the double determined points, x_{j2} is the second threshold measurement at each of the double determined points, and s_{2j} is the variance of the double determined thresholds at each of the points in the SF test for the reference population.

Figure 5-27. Formulas used for calculating global indices. Note each formula utilizes the known variances from the reference population to "weight" the significance of observed thresholds at each test point.

patient's island of vision lies below that of the reference population (ie, depressed). Mean deviation may represent many small depressions (overall depression) or significant loss in one part of the field and not in others (indicated by large values for PSD and CPSD, as discussed below).

Pattern standard deviation (PSD): a measure of the shape of the island of vision. The normal island of vision has a smooth, regular contour that drops off from the center to the periphery in an expected way. The contour, or shape, of the island of vision is represented by the calculated value of pattern standard deviation. PSD estimates the non-uniform (ie, local part of the deviation from normal) and may be thought of as the standard deviation of the numbers found in the total deviation array around the MD. If each point in the patient's visual field deviated from normal by the same amount (reflected in MD if different than zero), the PSD would be zero since the shape of that island of vision would parallel that of the reference population. If, however, a few points showed significant deviations, the spread of the deviations in the total deviation plot would be large, reflected in the PSD value. A large value indicates that the patient's island of vision does not have a smooth, regular contour; the larger the PSD, the more irregular the contour. Unlike MD, which is subject to diffuse effects, PSD is an indicator of scotomata within the field (assuming good patient reliability and

Figure 5-28. Fluctuation due to large spread in repeat measures of increased threshold in two points in the superior arcuate area. Points that are always double determined as part of the SF test are circled.

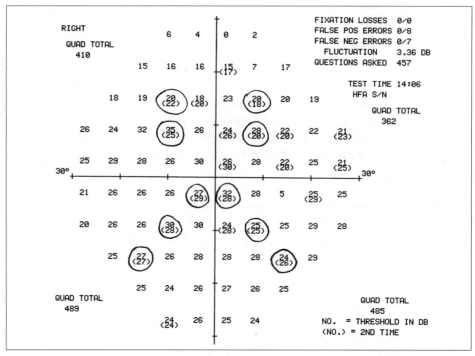

low variability), regardless of the overall height of the island of vision. PSD may also be thought of as a measure of how each test point compares to its surrounding points; points that are depressed (eg, within scotomata) will have threshold values significantly different from neighboring points and give rise to a large PSD.

Short-term fluctuation (SF): a measure of intratest variability, specifically referring to the difference between repeated threshold measurement at points within one test session. It is calculated by measuring threshold twice at 10 pre-determined points in the field (this is built into the Humphrey test software and is not unique to STATPAC) and then measuring the "spread" between the repeated measurements, averaging it over the field. Some older versions of the operating software require SF to be turned on and is not automatically calculated, in which case STATPAC will print the word "off" instead of a number. Later versions of the software default to SF on. High values of SF may indicate unreliability of patient responses (which would be reflected in the other reliability factors (eg, fixation losses, false positive responses, and false negative responses) or may represent increasing variability due to decreased sensitivity, either local or diffuse. Short-term fluctuation may be one of the most important aspects of a static threshold perimetric test—it has been shown that increasing fluctuation in one area of the visual field is inversely related to the sensitivity of that area and may be predictive of impending loss. Figure 5-28 is an example of increased fluctuation preceding the development of a superior arcuate defect. The 10 points that are always double-determined are circled. Note the large spread between repeated measures in two of them in the superior field (35 the first time, 25 the second, indicated by parentheses and 29 and 20), indicative of disturbance. This case is discussed in more detail in Chapter 6 (Figure 6-3).

Corrected pattern standard deviation (CPSD): PSD corrected for SF. As previously indicated, the PSD may be affected by high variability (ie, varying patient responses may make the contour of the island of vision appear irregular). STATPAC attempts to correct for this by factoring in the SF to the PSD and calculating the CPSD. If SF was not measured, STATPAC will print the word "off" instead of a number. This value represents the irregularity in the contour of the island of vision due to actual field loss, having removed the effects of patient variability. This number is the single most important indicator of the presence of scotomata within the field.

Visual field loss in glaucoma tends to occur in an asymmetric manner with respect to the horizontal meridian. Algorithms based on analysis of differences in clusters of mirror-image points across the horizontal meridian were developed during a natural history study of glaucoma. Åsman and Heijl developed an ana-

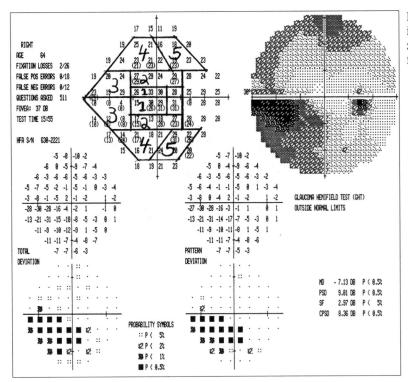

Figure 5-29. Clustering points into mirror-image groups above and below the horizontal meridian for the glaucoma hemifield test in STATPAC 2.

lytical algorithm designed to provide a similar analysis of differences across the horizontal meridian taking into account the known normal differences from the STATPAC database, including in that database all tests of all subjects, even the ones that were excluded because of unreliability (total 562 tests of 264 subjects). This has been termed the glaucoma hemifield test (GHT) and has been incorporated into STATPAC 2. Figure 5-29 shows how the test points are clustered into corresponding mirror-image areas above and below the horizontal axis. A test that does not demonstrate significant asymmetry between the paired cluster points will be labeled as "within normal limits;" clear asymmetric field defects will be identified as "outside normal limits," (Figure 5-30) as may shallow defects. "Borderline" results will be identified as such, and tests with abnormally high (Figure 5-31) or generalized reductions in sensitivity (Figure 5-32) can also be properly identified.

Fields demonstrating abnormally high sensitivity should be looked at carefully for a high false positive response rate. Even though the field shown in Figure 5-31 met the criteria for reliability, there are multiple white scotomata in the field and some impossible values in the field (55, 53, 47 40 dB). These are undoubtedly from false positive responses, but there were not enough catch trials for the rate to be abnormal. This patient had four out of 13 false positive responses; one more in the numerator or one less in the denominator and the rate would have met the 33% criteria to be indicated as unreliable.

The GHT will also report "outside normal limits" even if there is symmetrical loss across the horizontal if the loss exceeds the 0.5% limit. The GHT has been shown to be comparable to other methods of cross-meridional analysis in terms of sensitivity and specificity for detecting glaucomatous loss. Figure 5-33 is an excellent example of how subtle inferior loss can be highlighted in this patient with early glaucoma. Note how the apparent superior temporal "defect" on the graytone falls within normal limits for STATPAC.

Change in the Visual Field Over Time

A single visual field test is useful, sometimes essential, for making or confirming a diagnosis. However, the management of a chronic disease such as glaucoma relies upon the ability to determine the stability or deterioration of the visual field over time. In a test that is subject to significant variability in patient responses, sorting out true progression of defects from variability can be difficult. STATPAC and STATPAC 2 provide time analysis printouts designed to help make this distinction. The later versions of the operating soft-

Figure 5-30. Glaucoma hemifield test outside normal limits.

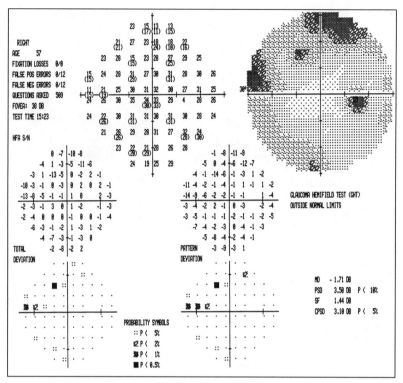

Figure 5-31. Abnormally high sensitivity indicated by the glaucoma hemifield test. Although the false positive catch trial rate was acceptable, there are a few points with "impossible" sensitivity. Mean deviations as high as that in this figure (+5.81) are usually due to false positive responses.

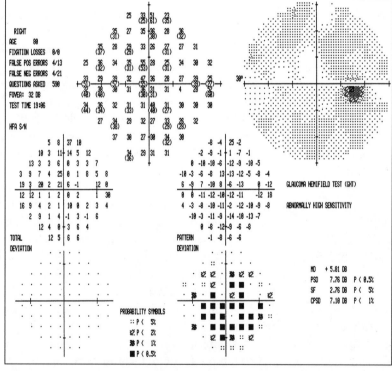

ware will automatically locate all of the tests from a selected patient (for one eye) provided the patient's name has been entered the same way each time. If the patient has been tested with 30-2 and 24-2 tests, the time analyses will be displayed for the points common to both grids.

Rather than taking single field printouts and spreading them over a desk or the floor to view them sequentially for change, STATPAC provides an overview printout (Figure 5-34), which can print the results of up to 16 tests on one page, displayed in chronological order. The printout contains the graytone, value table, total deviation probability plot, and pattern deviation probability plot for each test. Reliability and global indices

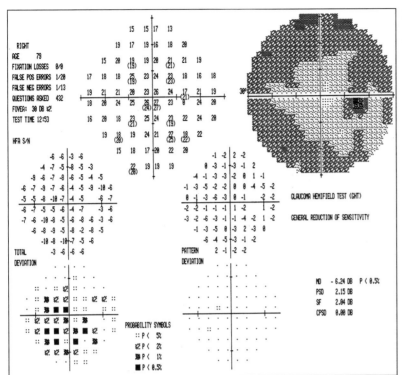

Figure 5-32. Generalized reduction in sensitivity identified by the glaucoma hemifield test.

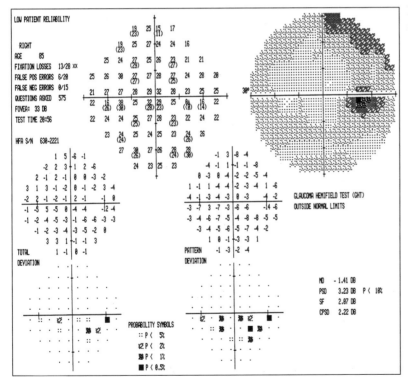

Figure 5-33. Subtle inferior defect emphasized by the glaucoma hemifield test.

are also displayed, and STATPAC 2 will print the results of the GHT across the top of each test. Results can be displayed for stimulus size III and V (stimulus V overview). Scanning down the page allows for a rapid survey of the field changes over time. Figure 5-34 is an example of a worsening inferior nasal step in a glaucoma patient.

The overview printout is essentially raw data. The change analysis printout (Figure 5-35, same patient as Figure 5-34) provides an analytical summary of visual field results from earliest to most recent, with up to

Figure 5-34. The STATPAC overview printout.

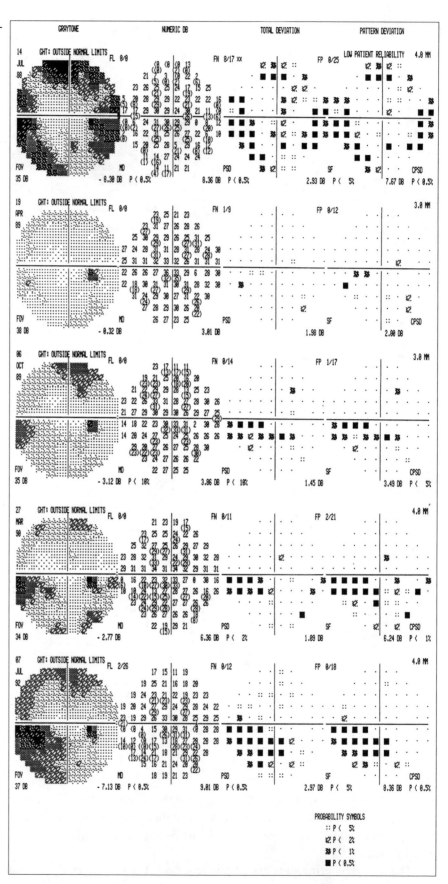

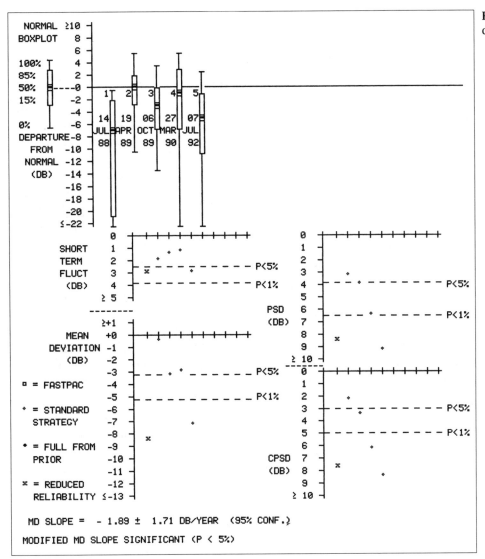

Figure 5-35. The STATPAC change analysis printout.

16 tests included. At the top of the printout is a modified histogram, known as the box plot. This summarizes the total deviation plot by listing the differences between the patient's measured thresholds and the age-corrected normals in order from smallest to largest. The scale on the left side of the plot lists possible departures from normal, ranging from greater than 10 dB above normal to more than 22 dB below normal, and a "normal" box derived from the normal database is shown to the left of the scale. The patient's best value (smallest depression or largest positive departure from normal) corresponds to the 100th percentile and is represented by the top line with a horizontal bar. The worst value, or the largest departure from age-corrected normal, is the first percentile and is represented by the bottom line with a horizontal bar. The top of the box represents the 85th percentile and the bottom represents the 15th. The median departure from normal (the 50th percentile) is represented by three horizontal bars in the middle of the box. Interpretation of the box plot considers the overall length of the box, the location of the box relative to "normal," the location of the median value, and the top and bottom end-point lines. Diffuse depression without localized defects will result in a normally shaped box printed lower down on the scale. A scotoma comprised of only a few points will have a relatively normal box with a long negative tail. Worsening scotomata will result in elongation of the box over time, usually with the entire box "sinking."

In addition to the box plot, the change analysis printout contains a change summary of the global indices—mean deviation, short-term fluctuation, pattern standard deviation, and corrected pattern standard deviation are plotted against time. The 5% and 1% limits for the reference population are represented by dashed lines. A patient value that falls below the 1% line, for example, would be expected in less than 1% of the reference population. A linear regression analysis on the mean deviation is performed if five or more tests have been conducted. The change in slope of the mean deviation over time (decibels/year) is displayed, and a comment is made as to whether or not the change is statistically significant.

STATPAC 2 adds a valuable time analysis printout for following glaucoma patients, known as the glaucoma change probability (Figure 5-36, same patient as Figures 5-34 and 5-35). It must be emphasized that this printout only applies to glaucoma patients (or suspects). Although the single-field analysis will compare the patient to the standard age-corrected normal database, the glaucoma change probability compares the patient to a population of "clinically stable" glaucoma patients, not age-corrected normals. The analysis uses the patient's first two tests as baseline and subsequent tests as follow-up; if only two tests have been performed, it will use the first as baseline and the second as follow-up. If five or more tests have been performed, the first test will be ignored if the mean deviation falls significantly below the regression line of the subsequent tests (P < 5%) to account for learning effects. This is the case in Figure 5-36—compare the overview printout (Figure 5-34) with the glaucoma change analysis. The analysis will not ignore unreliable tests, therefore a clinical judgment should be made to deselect from analysis tests that clearly showed the patient was inattentive, inexperienced, or otherwise unreliable. The printout contains the graytone and total deviation probability plots for each test, and the results of the glaucoma hemifield test appear above the graytone. For each of up to 14 follow-up tests, a point-by-point age-corrected change from baseline (not the previous test or the age-corrected normal thresholds) plot is provided. Positive numbers indicate improvement, negative indicates worsening, and zero means no change. The fourth column under follow-up indicates for each point the probability of the observed change occurring in the population of stable glaucoma patients. An open triangle indicates that the observed improvement would be expected in less than 5%, and a black triangle indicates worsening observed in less than 5% of the stable glaucoma patients. Change in mean deviation is provided under the change from baseline plot with the probability of observing that change in the reference population. A modified linear regression analysis is performed on mean deviation and plotted at the top of the printout next to the baseline examinations. The glaucoma change probability analysis has been shown to be comparable to "traditional intuitive criteria" for identifying visual deterioration at individual points within a visual field. The glaucoma change probability maps compare changes observed in the patient's visual fields with expected random variations that are seen in visual fields in glaucoma patients. Figure 5-37 is an example of a glaucoma patient with increasing cataract. Note general reduction in sensitivity and then improvement following cataract surgery in 1989.

Summary

The result of a visual field test is one aspect of a patient's visual function. Many disorders of the visual system affect the visual field in a known way, and a patient manifesting an abnormality in the visual field that matches a known pattern of loss will be given a certain diagnosis and perhaps be subjected to (life-long) treatment. It is of utmost importance to properly interpret the visual field results as to the presence or absence of abnormality, and this is usually accomplished by comparison of the patient to known normals. The STATPAC programs provide one mean for simplifying the performance of this comparison. It must be emphasized that an individual, even if manifesting departures from normal in a way expected in only a fraction of a percent of the normal population, may still be normal. In such a case, what happens to that individual's field over time becomes the driving force regarding therapy. Artifacts, normal variation, and congenital abnormalities of the optic nerve and other parts of the visual system all can result in visual field abnormalities resembling those found in treatable disease. All visual field data must be interpreted in light of the patient's overall clinical picture, and decisions regarding starting, changing, or stopping therapy should never be based on the results of a single examination. When doubt exists, it is best to repeat the examination for confirmation.

The results of a visual field examination are part of the care provided to a patient and as such, the results must be incorporated into the medical record. One never knows when one will need to explain the reason for

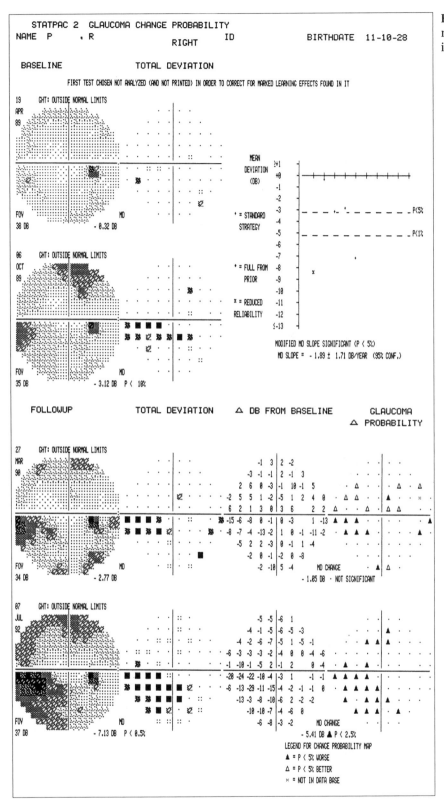

Figure 5-36. The STATPAC 2 glaucoma change probability plot showing progressive glaucomatous loss.

Figure 5-37. The STATPAC 2 glaucoma change probability plot showing diffuse loss of sensitivity due to progressive cataract and improvement following cataract surgery.

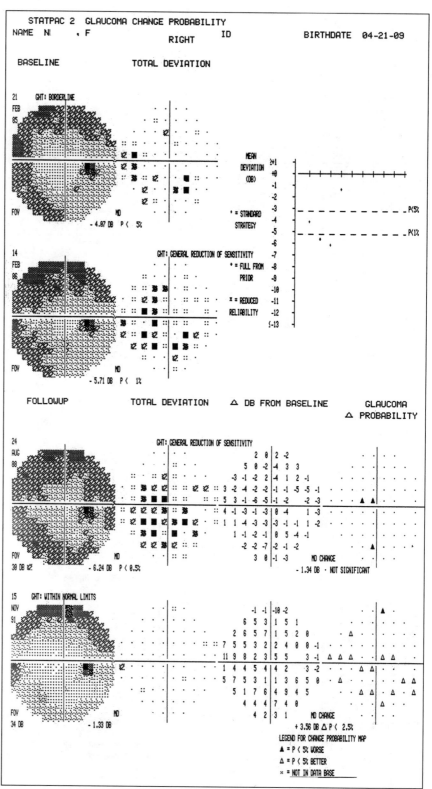

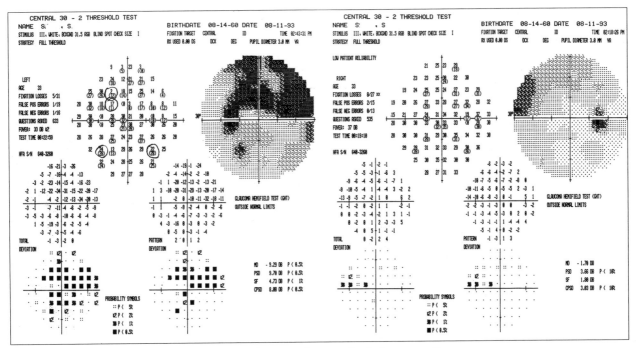

Figure 5-38. Visual fields from a patient with glaucoma for practice in interpretation.

a particular treatment or procedure. If the therapy was based partly on a visual field result, the interpretation of the result that prompted the therapy should be available in the record.

Figure 5-38 shows the visual fields from both eyes of a patient with glaucoma. Take a few moments and, using the material from this chapter, interpret the visual fields. Formulate a written interpretation as you would write it into the medical record of this patient. A suggested interpretation can be found at the end of this section. Remember, visual field interpretation, like almost everything that takes place in the practice of medicine, is fact-based opinion, and nothing more than that. Others may disagree with your interpretation but cannot find fault with treatment rendered that logically follows from that interpretation.

Suggested interpretation of visual fields shown in Figure 5-38:

OD: High fixation loss rate but otherwise reliable with a normal short-term fluctuation rate. Superior nasal depressions of moderate depth consistent with a nasal step compatible with early glaucoma.

OS: Reliable with high short-term fluctuation stemming from circled test points. A superior nerve fiber bundle defect and inferior paracentral loss of moderate depth are present. The field is consistent with moderate glaucomatous damage.

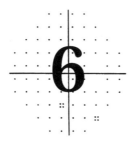

6

Visual Field Defects in Glaucoma

Adapted from Choplin N. Functional changes: psychophysical and electrophysiological testing. In: *Atlas of Ophthalmology*. Choplin NT, Lundy DC (eds). London: Martin Dunitz, LTD; 1998.

Introduction

Glaucoma is an optic neuropathy, and the disease is in reality a group of ocular conditions characterized by progressive loss of the nerve fibers that make up the optic nerve. The detection of nerve fiber loss and prevention of its development and progression is the ultimate goal of the ophthalmologist in the diagnosis and management of patients with glaucoma. At the present time, there is no proven reliable and consistent way to "count" optic nerve fibers, compare the "count" to known normals to determine the presence or absence of glaucomatous disease, and accurately determine if the "count" is changing over time. As axons are lost through the disease process, visual function declines in relation to the loss of fibers serving the region of loss. Therefore, tests of optic nerve function are integral to the management of glaucoma patients as an indirect measure of the number of axons remaining.

Visual Fields in Glaucoma

Of the subjective and objective tests currently available for diagnosing and following patients with glaucoma, visual field testing remains the mainstay. The use of automated perimetry has allowed the development of standardized tests for obtaining quantitative measurements. Such measurements can be compared to known normal values to determine the presence of abnormalities and can be followed over time for change. The statistical packages STATPAC, STATPAC II, and STATPAC for Windows have been developed to help in the interpretation of quantitative visual field data, both for determining abnormality in a single visual field examination and for determining the significance of observed changes in a series of visual fields measured over time. Portions of these packages, such as the glaucoma hemifield test and the glaucoma change probability plot, have been specifically developed to help the ophthalmologist interpret the visual field tests of glaucoma patients and suspects.

Damage to the visual field in glaucoma may occur in one of two ways or a combination of both, corresponding to observed patterns of axonal loss. Progressive optic nerve damage may occur diffusely, with concentric enlargement of the optic cup, progressive increase in the cup-to-disc ratio, and diffuse thinning of the neuro-retinal rim. The entire visual field may thus be diffusely affected, causing an increase in threshold for all points, which corresponds to a generalized reduction in sensitivity. This type of loss typifies the loss seen early in glaucoma associated with high intraocular pressure (ie, the "hyperbaric" type of glaucoma) and may be due to mechanical compression of axons as they pass through the lamina cribrosa. Damage may also occur in a more focal manner, with enlargement of the cup toward the superior and inferior poles of the disc with loss of portions of the neuro-retinal rim, resulting in nerve fiber bundle defects. This type of damage has been associated with "low-tension" glaucoma and may have a vascular etiology. The type of damage that occurs and the manner in which it progresses is not necessarily determined by the level of intraocular pressure, as there is considerable overlap in the intraocular pressure levels seen with both loss patterns. Although both patterns of loss have been observed in glaucoma patients, the mechanism by which each occurs and the role of intraocular pressure remains speculative at the present time. Both types of damage are seen late in all glaucomas, with extensive nerve fiber bundle defects and marked generalized loss of sensitivity.

The majority of visual field defects in glaucoma occur within the central 30°. Therefore, it is recommended that central 30° tests be used for following patients with glaucoma or who are at risk for developing glaucoma. It is also recommended that only threshold testing be done, with measurement of the short-term fluctuation. All of the examples in this chapter are the result of the 30-2 central test, which tests 76 points within the central 30° with a resolution of 6°. The points are offset from the axes by 3°, which allows localization of defects to one side of the axes or the other. Patients unable to complete the test because of the time required may be tested with the 24-2 threshold test, which eliminates some of the non-diagnostic peripheral points and still tests out to 30° nasally. The FASTPAC test strategy can also be used to reduce test time but may underestimate short-term fluctuation. Screening tests are not recommended for glaucoma patients because they do not measure fluctuation and may miss early defects in a patient whose entire hill of vision lies above that of an age-matched reference population. A new threshold algorithm, SITA (Swedish Interactive Thresholding Algorithm), discussed in Chapter 9, has recently been introduced. Since it seems to decrease test time without sacrificing accuracy, it may replace full-threshold testing as the preferred method for all visual field testing. This remains under investigation at the present time.

Generalized Reduction of Sensitivity in Glaucoma

Many factors acting on the field can produce diffuse loss, including incorrect refraction at the time of the test so that the patient was not properly focused on the interior of the bowl, media opacities such as cataract that reduce the amount of light entering the eye, small pupils, inattentiveness, false negative responses, and diffuse optic nerve damage. Optic nerve damage in glaucoma is often asymmetric with respect to the right and left eyes of a patient. Figure 6-1 shows the single field analysis printout from both eyes of a patient with asymmetric optic nerve damage. This set of visual fields illustrates a difference in mean sensitivity between the two eyes, indicative of asymmetric damage. The right eye shows no defect and the mean deviation when compared to age-corrected normals is +0.04 dB (decibels). The left eye shows no significant focal defect, but a mean deviation of -1.58 dB, indicating a mild overall reduction in sensitivity not only compared to the reference population but more importantly compared to the fellow eye. The intraocular pressure in the right eye was 16 mm Hg and was 23 mm Hg in the left. In addition, there was a mild increase in the cup-to-disc ratio in the left eye. This mild reduction in sensitivity in the left eye would not usually be considered clinically significant. However, when all the data is considered, it is consistent with mild diffuse depression and with early glaucomatous damage. Consequently, therapy was started in the left eye. This case illustrates the importance of comparing the fields from a patient's two eyes to each other in addition to the reference population.

Diffuse depression as the only glaucomatous defect may be easily detected with threshold testing, especially when statistical analysis is used to compare the patient's results to an age-corrected reference population. The patient illustrated in Figure 6-2 has long-standing open-angle glaucoma and has had recent uncon-

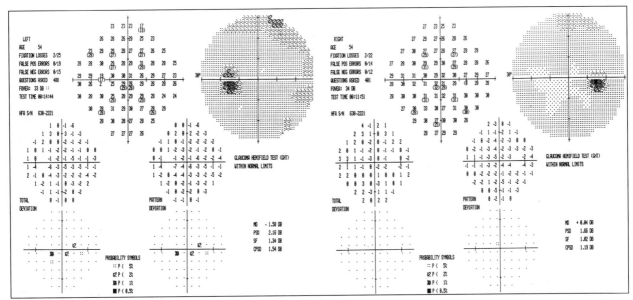

Figure 6-1. Visual fields from the right and left eyes of a patient with early asymmetric glaucomatous optic nerve damage. Note the difference in mean defect with an overall mild reduction in sensitivity in the left eye—the eye with the higher intraocular pressure and larger cup-to-disc ratio.

trolled intraocular pressure. He has been on maximum tolerated medical therapy and underwent argon laser trabeculoplasty when his pressure rose into the upper 20s. This visual field demonstrates diffuse depression of the visual field with a mean defect of -6.50 dB. The glaucoma hemifield test readily identifies the generalized reduction of sensitivity. The test was performed with the appropriate optical correction following dilation of the pupils, including the full +3.25 add, and the optical media was clear. Review of the disc photographs showed a gradual increase in the cup-to-disc ratio over time, corresponding to the gradual diffuse loss of sensitivity.

The results of psychophysical tests, such as visual field testing, are subject to a certain degree of variability. This test-retest variability in threshold perimetry is measurable, has known normal values, and has clinical significance. It has been shown that as retinal sensitivity decreases, the variability of threshold in that region increases. It has also been shown that increasing fluctuation may precede the development of a visual field defect, thus giving its measurement particular clinical importance. Figure 6-3 illustrates a patient with angle-recession glaucoma with intraocular pressure in the low 30s. The field demonstrates diffuse depression and an eyelid artifact (the globe was enophthalmic due to an orbital floor fracture so that the upper lid was ptotic), but more importantly an increased short-term fluctuation (SF) value of 3.36, expected in less than 2% of the reference population. The high value is derived from two points in the superior arcuate area (circled): one showing measurements of 35 dB and 25 dB, and the other 28 dB and 20 dB. These large differences in repeat measurements (10 dB and eight decibels respectively) point to disturbed portions of the visual field that will most likely go on to develop paracentral and arcuate defects. The short-term fluctuation measurement is very important in evaluating glaucoma patients and glaucoma suspects, particularly since increasing fluctuation may be the earliest sign of glaucomatous optic nerve damage.

Early Focal Loss in Glaucoma

The retinal nerve fiber layer is constructed in such a manner that no axons cross the horizontal midline and defects associated with optic neuropathies (such as glaucoma) tend to localize to one side of the horizontal or the other. Fibers from the macula run into the temporal aspect of the nerve as the papulomacular bundle; axons peripheral to the fovea have to arch over this bundle to reach the nerve and insert in the poles of the disc. Fibers from the nasal retina are radially oriented with respect to the disc. It is the loss of axons

Figure 6-2. An example of diffuse loss of sensitivity in a patient with open-angle glaucoma. The patient has clear optical media and was tested with dilated pupils and the appropriate optical correction.

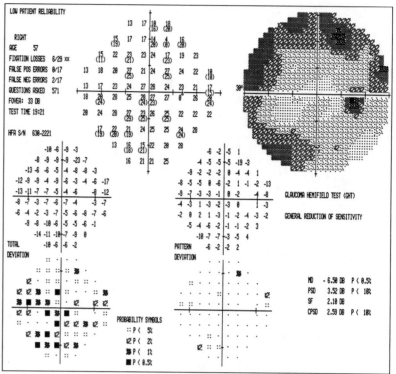

Figure 6-3. This visual field from a patient with increased intraocular pressure shows diffuse loss of sensitivity and an increase in short-term fluctuation, indicated by the large spread in repeat threshold measures in the two circled points. This patient is likely to develop a visual field defect in this disturbed portion of the visual field.

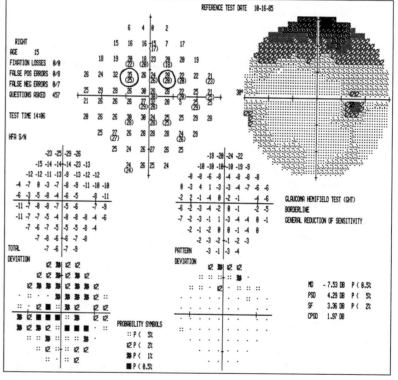

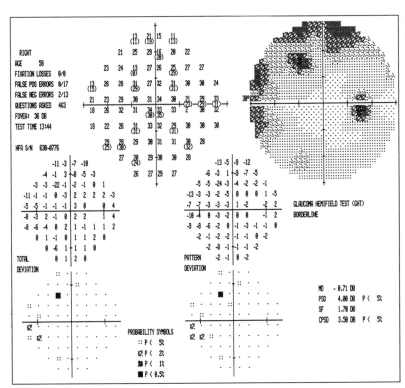

Figure 6-4. Isolated superior paracentral scotoma in a patient with early glaucoma.

that results in the visual field defects observed in glaucoma. The size and shape of these defects are determined by the location and extent of the nerve fiber loss; loss of arcuate fibers on the temporal side of the disc will result in arcuate defects, and loss of radial fibers on the nasal side will result in wedge-shaped defects. Of course, due to the optics of the eye, the location of the visual field defect will be reversed superior to inferior and nasal to temporal with respect to the location of the nerve fiber loss (eg, a defect in inferotemporal nerve fibers will result in a superonasal visual field defect).

Isolated paracentral defects occur as the initial glaucoma defect in about 40% of patients. Other early manifestations of glaucoma damage include arcuate defects, nasal steps, and temporal wedge defects. The patient illustrated in Figure 6-4 shows an isolated defect in the superior paracentral region measuring 22 dB below normal. Note the wide fluctuation in repeat measurements of this point (13 dB then 0 dB). Untreated intraocular pressure was in the upper 20s in this eye.

Figure 6-5 shows mild asymmetric loss in the inferior hemifield. The pattern deviation shows a small inferior arcuate scotoma. Note also how STATPAC highlights the significance of the magnitude of this defect in this portion of the visual field, indicating that these threshold measurements would be expected in less than 0.5% of the age-matched reference population. Although other more peripheral areas have similar threshold measurements (hence the same appearance on the graytone plot), STATPAC indicates that these values are common in the normal population and are not defects. The asymmetric nature of the damage with respect to the horizontal midline is further emphasized by the abnormal glaucoma hemifield test.

Figures 6-6 through 6-10 are additional examples of early glaucomatous defects. Figure 6-6 shows an inferior arcuate scotoma in the absence of any diffuse loss; note how the total deviation plot and the pattern deviation plot are virtually identical. Figure 6-7 illustrates an inferior arcuate scotoma and inferior nasal step, again in the absence of diffuse loss. These defects indicate early damage to the superior pole of the optic nerve and are both parts of the same nerve fiber bundle. If damage continues in this area, these defects will coalesce to form a complete nerve fiber bundle defect. Figure 6-8 is a moderately advanced superior nasal step in a patient with juvenile glaucoma. Figure 6-9 is a well-developed inferior arcuate scotoma in a patient with end-stage glaucoma in the fellow eye. Note that this defect does not break through to the nasal periphery. Finally, Figure 6-10 illustrates temporal wedge defects. These defects, which are wedge shaped due to the radial orientation of the nerve fibers on the nasal side of the disc, occur as the initial defects in glaucoma less than 3% of the time.

Figure 6-5. Early inferior arcuate scotoma unmasked by STATPAC.

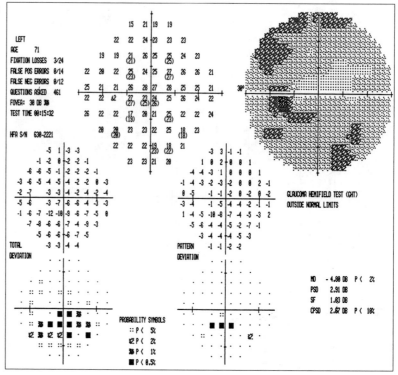

Figure 6-6. Isolated inferior arcuate scotoma without diffuse loss.

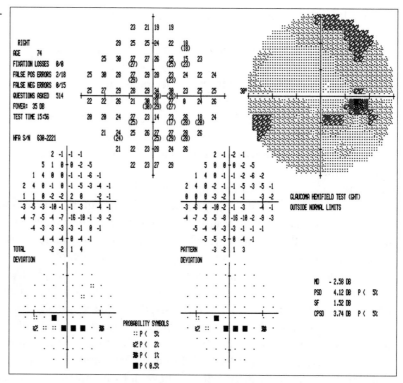

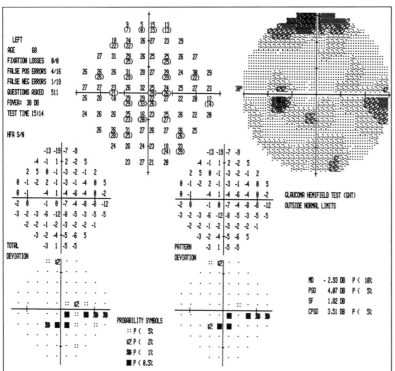

Figure 6-7. Paracentral defects and inferior nasal step within the same nerve fiber bundle.

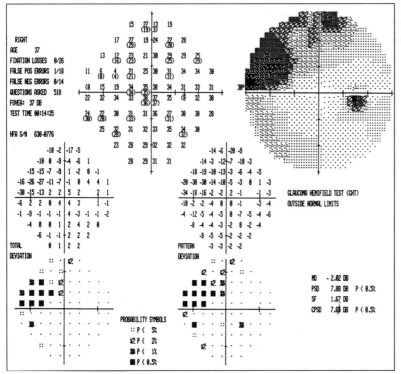

Figure 6-8. Moderately advanced superior nasal step in a patient with juvenile glaucoma.

Figure 6-9. Inferior arcuate scotoma not breaking out to nasal periphery.

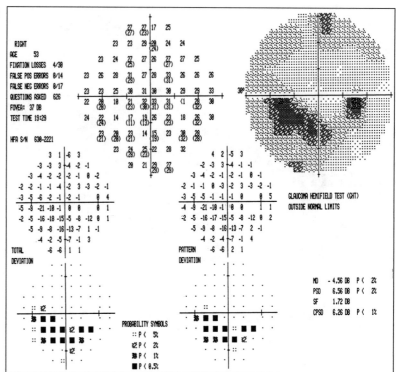

Advanced Glaucomatous Visual Field Loss

Loss of larger bundles of nerve fibers results in more extensive visual field defects. Figure 6-11 illustrates an almost complete nerve fiber bundle defect resulting from extension of the cup to the inferior pole of the disc and loss of rim at the 6:30 position. Figure 6-12 shows complete nerve fiber bundle defects, OS greater than OD, in a patient with open-angle glaucoma and loss of rim tissue inferiorly in both eyes. The patient in Figure 6-13 has moderately advanced glaucoma damage and shows a "double arcuate" scotoma, consisting of superior and inferior nerve fiber bundle defects. Note the inferior defect is greater than the superior. Just as damage is often asymmetric with respect to the two eyes of a patient, it is often asymmetric with respect to the horizontal midline. As damage continues and visual field loss progresses, an entire hemifield may become involved, resulting in an altitudinal defect, as illustrated in Figure 6-14. This patient has low-tension glaucoma and temporal arteritis. Although she never had an episode of ischemic optic neuropathy, it is possible that this sort of damage is partially caused by poor optic nerve blood flow and ischemia. Figure 6-15 shows far advanced glaucomatous loss in a patient with low-tension glaucoma, with a small central island and temporal field remaining. Finally, Figure 6-16 is the visual field of a patient with end-stage glaucomatous visual field loss who has reduced central acuity due to the optic neuropathy. This patient has juvenile-onset glaucoma and became symptomatic as his loss extended into his central field. This was his visual field upon presentation when intraocular pressure was in the 50s. Following filtering surgery and stabilization of his pressure in the low teens, his visual acuity improved from 20/70 to 20/25 and some portions of this field improved.

Progression of Glaucomatous Visual Field Loss

Uncontrolled glaucoma may show progressive visual field loss in a number of ways as the reserve of nerve fibers is used up and as fibers continue to be lost. Patients initially having no defects may first manifest diffuse loss of sensitivity, increased short-term fluctuation, or begin to develop focal defects. Continued loss may result in further diffuse loss in sensitivity, widening and deepening of existing focal defects as fur-

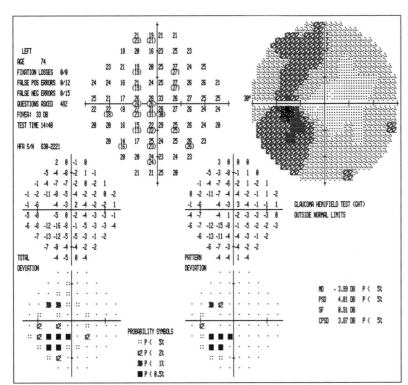

Figure 6-10. Temporal wedge defects in a patient with early glaucoma.

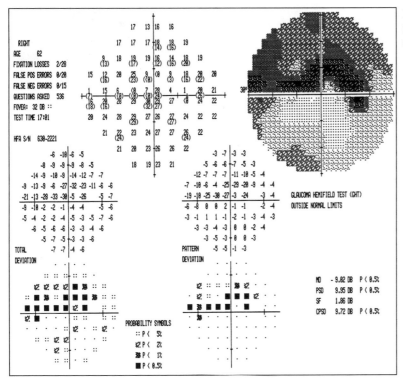

Figure 6-11. Incomplete superior nerve fiber bundle defect characterized by an arcuate scotoma and superior nasal step.

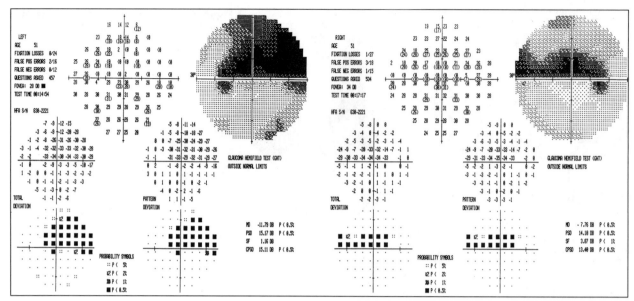

Figure 6-12. Complete nerve fiber bundle defects, left eye greater than right, from both eyes of a glaucoma patient.

Figure 6-13. The "double arcuate" scotoma, consisting of nerve fiber bundle defects at both poles of the disc.

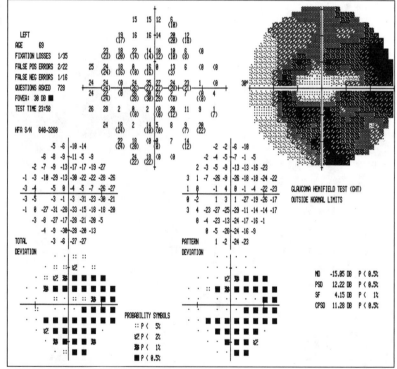

ther axons within a bundle become involved, or develop new defects in other portions of the field as new bundles become damaged. Of course, any combination of the above changes may be observed.

Figure 6-17 is an example of the development of diffuse loss of sensitivity over a seven-year period in an African-American man with elevated intraocular pressure. Although his pressure had been treated from the beginning, it became uncontrolled at various times during this follow-up period and he required laser treatment. The glaucoma change probability plot shows how he gradually lost sensitivity diffusely throughout the field in a manner not expected in the age-corrected reference population of stable glaucoma patients. Note that over this period of time, the mean deviation increased from approximately one to 6.5 dB. This is particularly evident in the graph of mean deviation in the upper right of the figure. Review of optic disc pho-

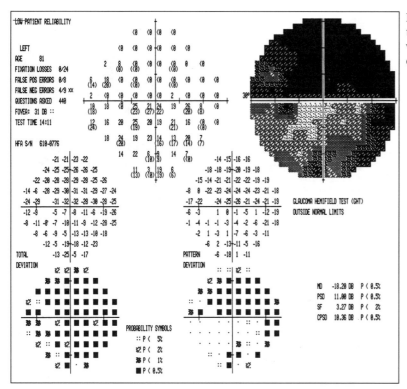

Figure 6-14. An altitudinal defect involving the entire superior hemifield of a patient with low-tension glaucoma and extensive optic nerve damage.

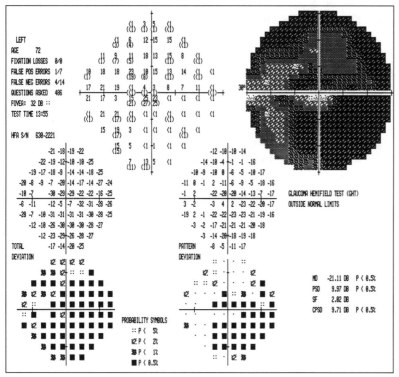

Figure 6-15. Far advanced glaucomatous damage with a small central island and relatively better sensitivity temporally remaining.

Figure 6-16. End-stage visual field in a patient presenting with intraocular pressure in excess of 50 mm Hg and far advanced glaucomatous optic neuropathy.

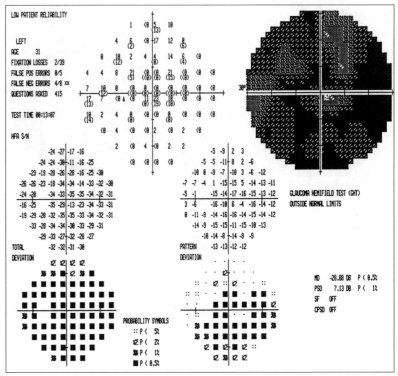

tographs obtained during this period of time showed a gradual enlargement of the cup-to-disc ratio, consistent with this diffuse change in the visual field. The last field in this series is the same as Figure 6-2.

Initial visual field loss may be represented by small focal defects. Figure 6-18 shows the development of a reproducible superior nasal step in the right eye of a glaucoma suspect over a four-year period.

Fields initially with defects may show the development of new defects. Figure 6-19 is a series of fields in a patient with open-angle glaucoma showing completion of an inferior nerve fiber bundle defect as well as the development of new defects in the superior field. Part of the diffuse change in the latter fields is due to the development of cataract.

Visual fields may progress by widening and deepening of single nerve fiber bundle defects. The series of visual fields in Figure 6-20 is from the patient in Figure 6-11. Initially the field showed mild superonasal loss and then the patient developed disturbances in the superior arcuate area. These coalesced and extended over time to involve almost the entire bundle of axons and a good portion of the superior field. Another example of extension of an existing defect and development of a new defect os seen in Figure 6-21.

The series of visual fields in Figure 6-22 was obtained from the fellow eye of the same patient in Figure 6-16. Note the gradual enlargement of the superior nasal step. The intraocular pressure on maximum tolerated medical therapy was in the mid 20s, and the patient has undergone filtering surgery in this eye.

Figure 6-23 is the series of visual fields of the patient in Figure 6-15. The initial inferior nerve fiber bundle defect has extended and the patient has developed new defects in the superior hemifield. The statistical software plots the mean deviation over time as a graph on the right side of the top of the printout and performs statistical tests for significant change over time. This series shows a steady decline of about 0.8 dB per year. This is considered statistically significant.

Finally, Figure 6-24 illustrates the extension of a dense superior nerve fiber bundle defect to a complete altitudinal defect over a six-year period.

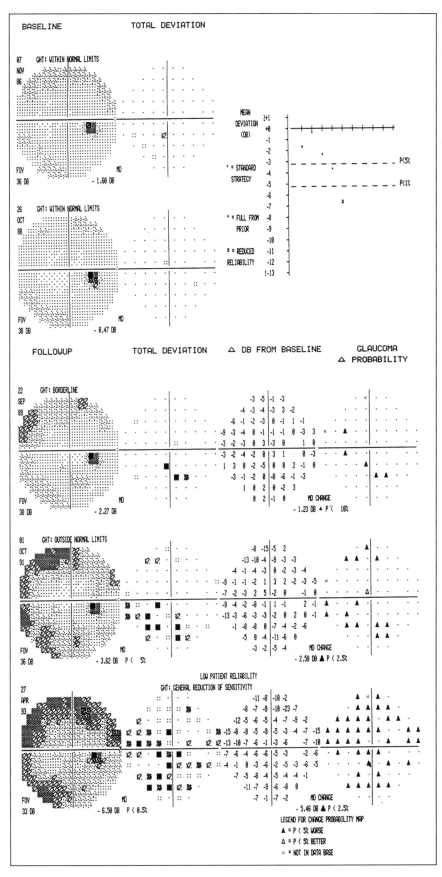

Figure 6-17. Diffuse loss of sensitivity developing over a seven-year period.

Figure 6-18. Development of a reproducible superior nasal step in the right eye of a glaucoma suspect over a four-year period. There is also some mild depression in the superior arcuate area. Treatment was instituted based on this visual field.

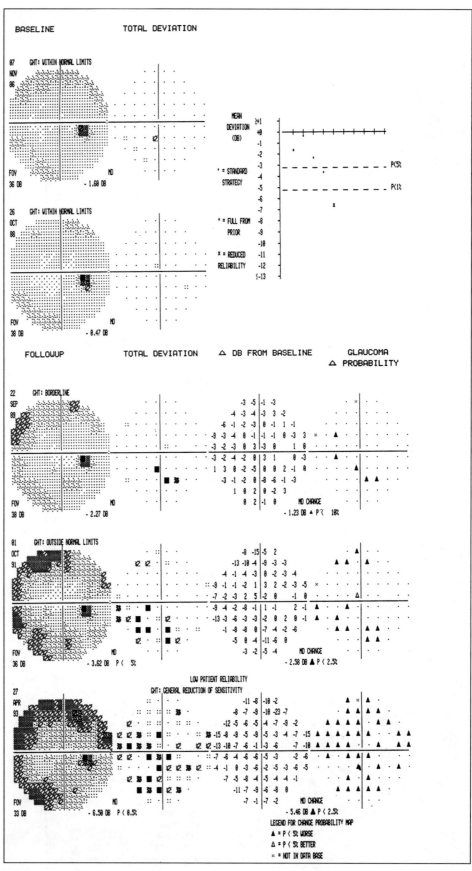

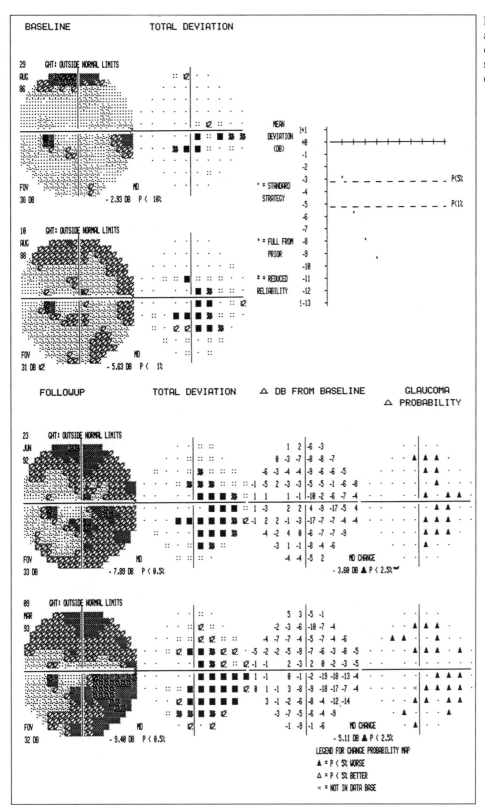

Figure 6-19. Progression of an inferior defect and development and extension of a superior defect over a seven-year period.

Figure 6-20. Development and extension of a superior defect to an almost complete nerve fiber bundle defect.

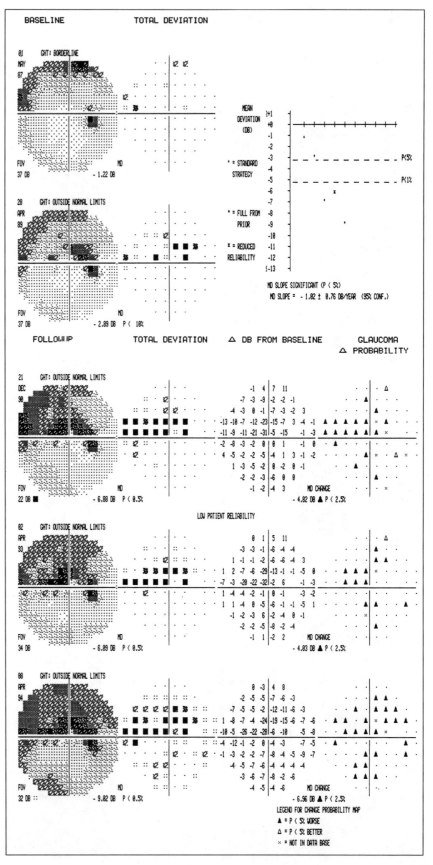

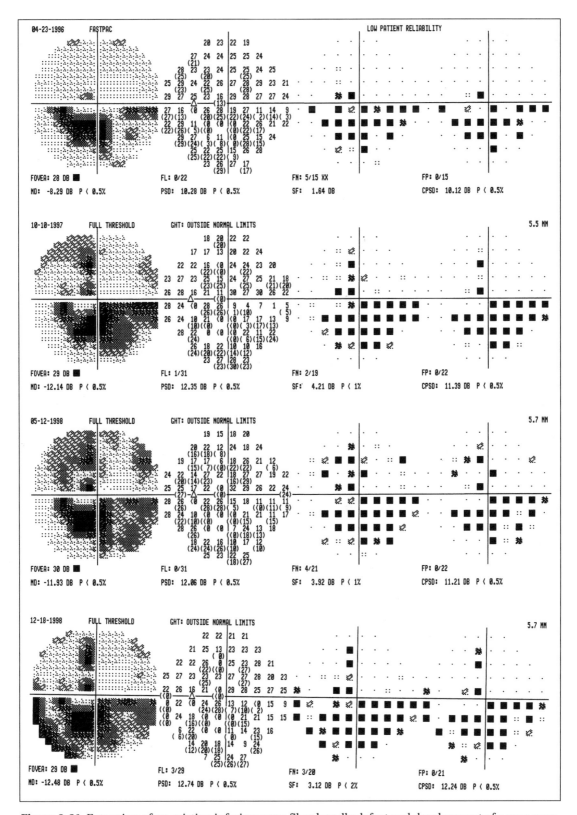

Figure 6-21. Extension of an existing inferior nerve fiber bundle defect and development of a new superior defect over a two-year period in a glaucoma patient.

Figure 6-22. Extension of a superior nasal step by widening and broadening.

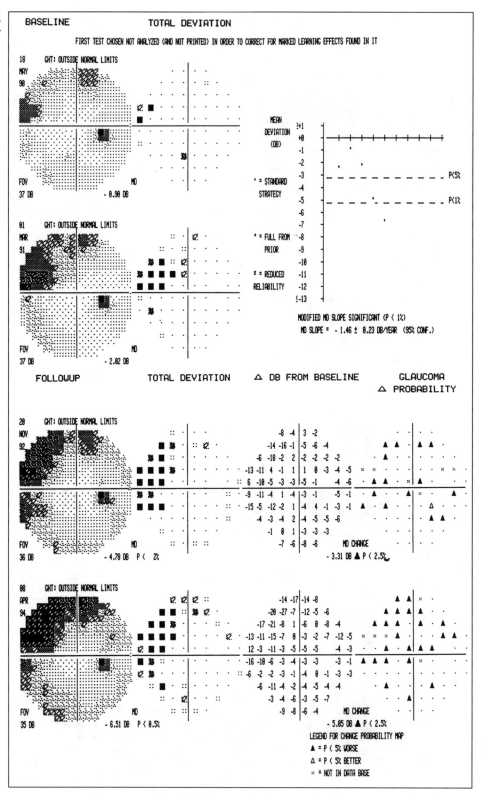

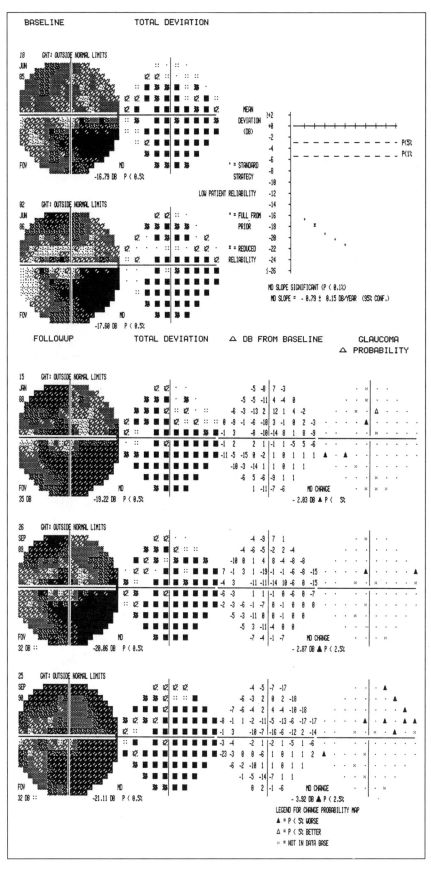

Figure 6-23. Extension of an inferior nerve fiber bundle defect and development of new defects in the superior hemifield.

Figure 6-24. Completion of an altitudinal defect over a six-year period in a patient with low-tension glaucoma and small vessel ischemic disease attributable to temporal arteritis.

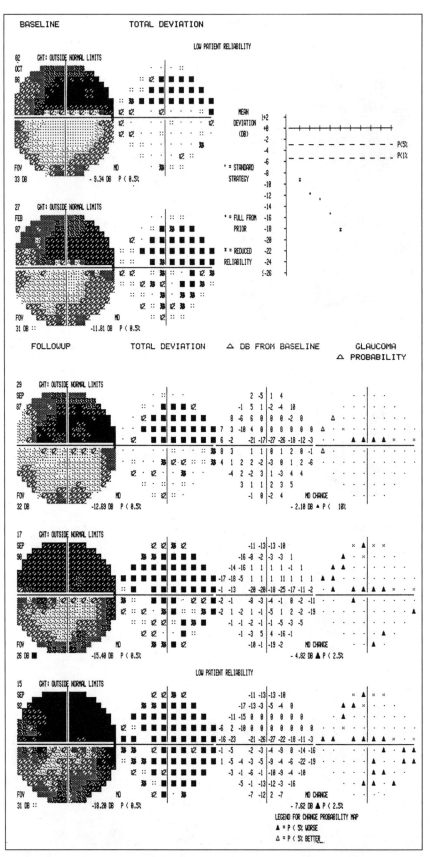

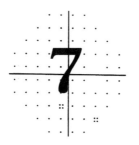

Visual Field Defects in Neuro-Ophthalmology as Measured by the Humphrey Field Analyzer

Introduction

The visual field examination is an important component in the evaluation of the patient with neurologic conditions affecting the visual system. Perimetry can be used to detect and quantify visual field abnormalities as well as to follow the patient's response to treatment. It can confirm the presence of a visual defect in a symptomatic patient when other measures of visual function (such as visual acuity) fail to do so. Patients with no visual complaints, such as those with headache syndromes, may show visual field defects that assist in diagnosis. The pattern of visual field loss may pinpoint the location of the problem in the visual pathways, which can help the clinician in selecting the proper neurodiagnostic studies. This chapter discusses the role of the Humphrey perimeter in the clinical evaluation of the neuro-ophthalmic patient.

Neuro-Anatomy

An understanding of the neuro-anatomy of the visual system guides the clinician facing a neuro-ophthalmic problem to proper visual field test selection, as well in the interpretation of the findings. At times, the patterns of visual field loss can precisely localize the causative lesion. These patterns are the result of the course that visual neurons take as they traverse from the retina to the occipital cortex. A brief review of the visual pathways will be made to help the reader understand the power of the visual field in the localization of lesions of the afferent visual system. Discussion of the anatomy will start in the eye and follow the course of the visual neurons to the brain; the examples shown in this chapter will be presented in the same "front-to-back" progression.

The neurons that comprise the optic nerve originate in the ganglion cells in the retina. Axons from the ganglion cells course toward the optic disc in the nerve fiber layer. Fibers originating in the inferior retina (subserving the superior visual field) enter the disc inferiorly, while fibers originating in the superior retina (subserving the inferior visual field) enter the disc superiorly. Furthermore, neurons originating temporal to the fovea (subserving the nasal visual field) enter the optic disc at the superior and inferior poles, bending around the macula in arcuate bundles. Axons originating nasal to the fovea (subserving the temporal visual field) enter the disc on the nasal and temporal sides, with the maculopapular bundle entering the disc on its temporal side. Lesions of the optic disc therefore produce visual field defects that do not cross the horizontal meridian. Nasal steps, arcuate bundle defects, and temporal wedge defects are the primary visual field defects found in diseases affecting the optic nerve head.

The neurons enter the optic disc in bundles that pass through the pores in the lamina cribrosa. As they traverse the optic nerve on their path toward the optic chiasm, the macular fibers move to a more central location in the nerve. The axons tend to maintain the temporal-nasal and superior-inferior relationship that began in the retina. Since large numbers of neurons carry macular information, lesions of the optic nerve tend to produce unilateral central field defects, but other patterns are commonly seen.

At the optic chiasm, axons that originated nasal to the fovea cross to the opposite side while those from the temporal side continue in their path toward the lateral geniculate ganglion without crossing. In this hemidecussation, the superonasal fibers bend anteriorly into the opposite optic nerve before resuming their generally posterior direction (von Willebrand's knee).

After leaving the optic chiasm, the axons that originated in the retinal ganglion cells continue posteriorly in the optic tract until reaching the lateral geniculate body in the basal ganglia. There, they synapse with the cells whose axons are destined for the occipital cortex. These axons fan out in the optic radiations. Some of the inferior fibers bend around the temporal horn of the lateral ventricle into the temporal lobe on their way to the inferior portion of the occipital pole. These fibers are known as Meyer's loop. The superior fibers take a more direct route through the parietal lobe, finally reaching the superior portion of the occipital pole. Macular fibers project onto the tip and over the outer surface of the occipital cortex, while the fibers serving the peripheral visual field terminate on either side of the calcarine fissure on the medial surface of the occipital lobes.

Notice that after leaving the optic chiasm, the fibers from one side no longer represent that side's eye, but rather the visual space on the opposite side. Lesions in the visual pathways behind the chiasm produce field defects on one side of both eyes. Known as homonymous hemianopias, these defects do not cross the vertical meridian. As they course posteriorly, fibers representing adjacent visual space are closer together, therefore visual field defects tend to become more alike in each eye (congruous) as the causative lesion gets closer to the occipital lobe.

Optic Disc-Based Field Loss

Glaucoma is the most common and best known disease that causes disc-based visual field loss. Visual field defects arising from glaucoma are discussed extensively in Chapter 6. A variety of neuro-ophthalmic disorders are also associated with optic disc injury. Congenital anomalies, optic disc drusen, inflammatory disease, tumors, and ischemic disorders can all affect the nerve fibers entering the optic disc and cause visual field abnormalities. Automated perimetry can detect these field defects, quantify them, and allow for determining the effectiveness of therapy.

Since the retinal nerve fibers are arranged in a manner such that they do not cross the horizontal meridian, optic disc-based field loss tends to occur either above or below a horizontal line drawn through fixation. When they occur both above and below the horizontal meridian, the defects above usually do not "match up" with the defects found below. The most commonly recognized defects are nasal steps, arcuate scotomas, and altitudinal defects. Temporal wedge defects and central or paracentral scotomas can also be found in optic disc-based visual field loss.

Optic Disc Drusen

Optic disc drusen are accumulations of a hyaline-like material within the optic disc anterior to the lamina cribrosa. Patients with disc drusen are usually asymptomatic and have normal visual acuity. Optic disc drusen are fairly common, occurring in about 1% of the population. They are frequently discovered on routine ophthalmologic examination; buried drusen may cause optic disc elevation and are a common cause of

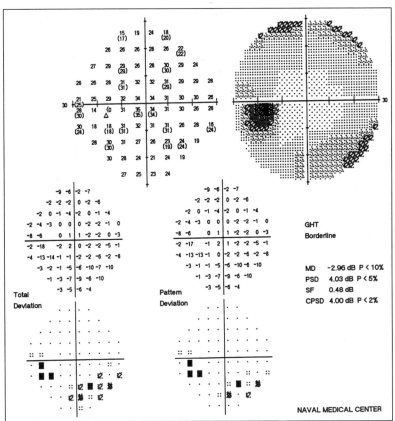

Figure 7-1a. An example of a visual field from an eye with optic disc drusen, showing inferior visual field loss.

pseudopapilledema. Figure 7-1 shows the visual field (a) and ultrasound examination (b) of a patient with optic disc drusen. Figure 7-2 is a central 30-2 field from the left eye of a patient with visible disc drusen. This field shows a superior nasal step with shallow defects in both the inferior and superior Bjerrum areas. The abnormality extending temporally from the blind spot is a temporal wedge defect. Figure 7-3 is the visual field from the right eye of the same patient in Figure 7-2. The patient has a relative afferent pupillary defect associated with this severe visual field loss. Visual field loss in patients with disc drusen can assume any of the patterns described above for disc-based loss, with nasal steps, arcuate scotomas, and temporal wedge defects being the most common. Central scotomas can occur but are not common.

PAPILLEDEMA

Papilledema is a result of increased intracranial pressure. In papilledema, the optic disc is swollen, often with congestion of the retinal veins and peripapillary hemorrhages, as is seen in Figure 7-4. A variety of conditions can cause increased intracranial pressure, including brain tumors, meningitis, encephalitis, intracerebral hemorrhage, and subarachnoid hemorrhage. A common cause is pseudotumor cerebri, a condition of elevated intracranial pressure of unknown etiology. Visual field abnormalities in patients with papilledema may be the result of the underlying disorder causing increased intracranial pressure, but may also occur as a result of the chronically swollen nerve.

In early papilledema, antegrade axoplasmic flow is impeded and axonal swelling occurs. Later, extracellular edema is also found. Visual field abnormalities in acute papilledema are usually limited to an increase in the size of the blind spot. With time, the circulation of the optic disc may be compromised, resulting in disc-based visual field loss, which in many cases is reversible with treatment of the increased intracranial pressure. When optic atrophy occurs, full recovery is usually not expected. The visual field in Figure 7-5 is a central 30-2 threshold exam of the right eye of a 38-year-old woman with pseudotumor cerebri. It is a reliable exam, based on the catch trials, and shows classic disc-based field loss with an inferior nasal step and an inferior temporal wedge defect. Figure 7-6 is a central 30-2 threshold exam in a 41-year-old woman with

Figure 7-1b. The drusen can be seen as the bright reflections (arrows) overlying the optic nerve on the ultrasound examination.

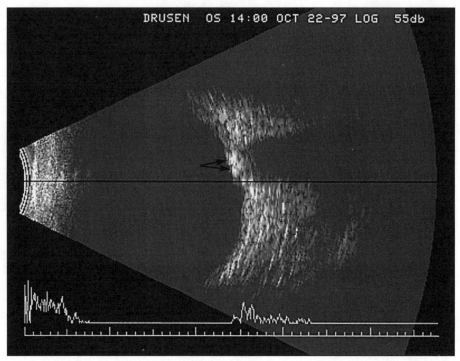

Figure 7-2. Threshold exam of the left eye from a patient with optic disc drusen.

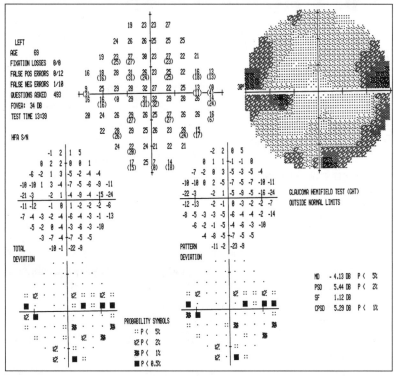

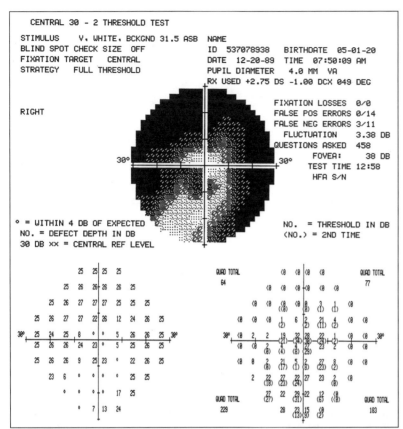

Figure 7-3. Stimulus V threshold exam of the fellow eye of the patient in Figure 7-2.

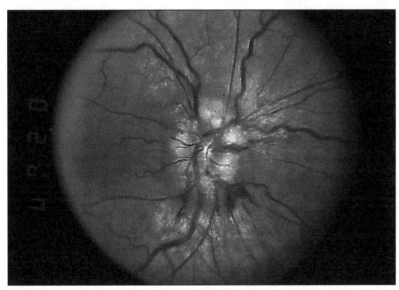

Figure 7-4. Optic nerve photograph from a patient with acute papilledema.

Figure 7-5. Threshold exam from a patient with pseudotumor cerebri and papilledema.

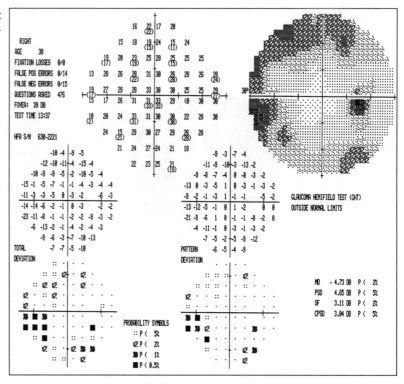

pseudotumor cerebri. Note the increased blind spot. There is a shallow paracentral depression that is not deep enough to be revealed by the graytone display. Shallow depressions in the superior arcuate area are also present. Treatment with acetazolamide resulted in normalization of the intracranial pressure and resolution of field defects, as seen in Figure 7-7.

ANTERIOR ISCHEMIC OPTIC NEUROPATHY

Anterior ischemic optic neuropathy (AION) is an optic nerve disorder related to decreased circulation to the nerve associated with acute loss of vision. Nonarteritic AION and giant cell arteritis are the most common causes of AION, but a number of other diseases may also cause it, including sickle cell disease and the collagen vascular disorders. Patients with AION have painless loss of vision over a period of several hours to days. Visual acuity is usually decreased, often severely. Disc-based visual field loss occurs, with altitudinal defects being most common. The central 30-2 threshold exam of a 55-year-old man with a three-day history of blurred vision in his left eye is shown in Figure 7-8. His acuity at the time of the field exam was 20/40 and he had pale disc edema. Because the patient was seeing so few of the stimulus presentations with the standard size III stimulus, the technician changed the stimulus size to a Goldmann size V and restarted the test. Note the dense superior altitudinal field defect. Because STATPAC does not include age-related normal values for the size V stimulus, the usual single field analysis printout is not available, and a three-in-one display is used instead. The numeric values on the lower right-hand side are the measured threshold values. The "quad total" is the sum of all the threshold values for a quadrant, allowing a quick assessment of the amount of loss of retinal sensitivity in each quadrant. The numeric values on the lower left-hand side are calculated values based on the visual field profile constructed from the central reference level. Values that lie within 4 decibels (dB) of expected are labeled with a "0;" all other points are labeled with a value that is the difference between the expected value and the measured threshold: in the defect depth display, low numbers are "good" and high numbers "bad."

Figure 7-9 is a central 30-2 threshold exam from a 59-year-old man who developed an acute anterior ischemic optic neuropathy following coronary artery bypass surgery. This patient had preservation of central acuity; the visual field shows an inferior altitudinal defect with central sparing. Note the normal foveal threshold level. The glaucoma hemifield test is outside normal limits, as expected in the presence of an altitudinal defect.

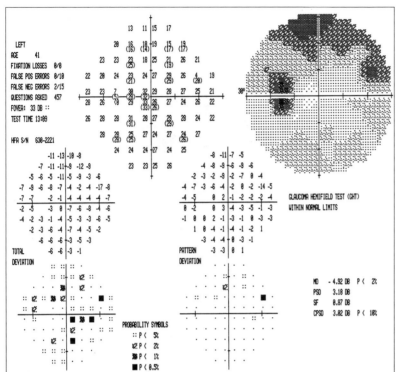

Figure 7-6. Threshold exam from a patient with pseudotumor cerebri and papilledema.

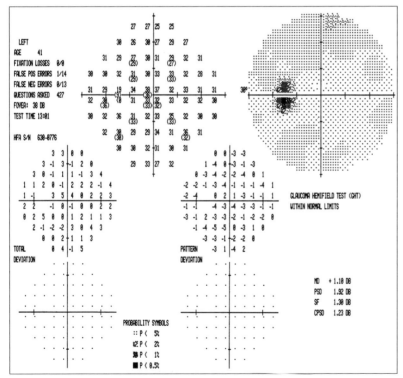

Figure 7-7. Threshold exam from the same patient as Figure 7-6, following therapy.

Figure 7-8. Stimulus V threshold exam from a patient with nonarteritic anterior ischemic optic neuropathy.

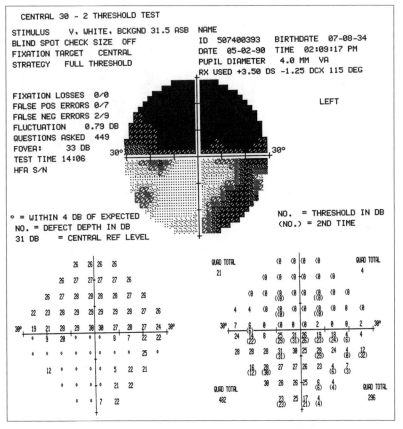

Figure 7-9. Threshold exam from a patient with anterior ischemic optic neuropathy following coronary artery bypass surgery.

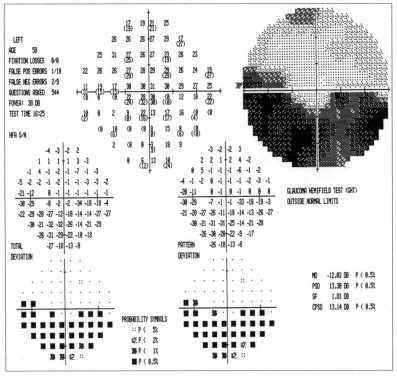

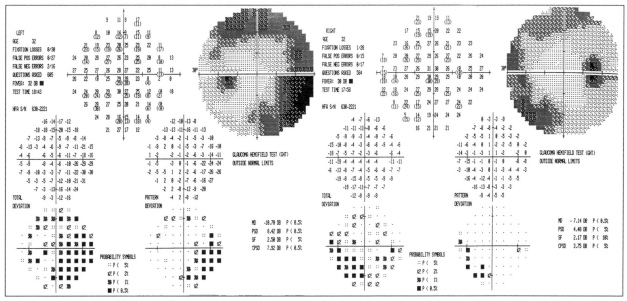

Figure 7-10. Threshold exam of both eyes from a patient with optic neuritis.

Optic Nerve Lesions

Optic nerve lesions can produce a variety of visual field defects. Axons subserving adjacent areas of the visual field tend to lie near each other, with macular fibers concentrated in the center of the optic nerve. Compressive lesions may cause relatively more dysfunction in the central part of the nerve and are more often associated with central scotomas. Localized lesions in the nerve can cause the same defects found in disc-based field loss, as well as central and paracentral scotomas. Focal defects may cross the horizontal meridian in optic nerve lesions. While lesions of one optic nerve do not affect the field in the opposite eye, many causes of optic nerve disease can affect both eyes.

OPTIC NEURITIS

One of the common optic nerve diseases is optic neuritis. While there are many causes of optic neuritis, its association with multiple sclerosis is the strongest. Optic neuritis causes visual loss that progresses over a period of several days to a week or so. Visual acuity is usually decreased, there is a loss of color vision, and an afferent pupillary defect (Marcus-Gunn pupil) develops on the affected side. Pain on eye movement is a common association. Optic neuritis may be retrobulbar or involve the optic disc, in which case it is known as papillitis. In the clinical variant of optic neuritis known as papillitis, disc swelling that is indistinguishable with papilledema is present. If the episode of optic neuritis is the patient's first, the eye's appearance may be normal ("the patient sees nothing and the doctor sees nothing"). It is not unusual to see visual field abnormalities in the asymptomatic fellow eye of a patient with optic neuritis.

Figure 7-10 is a central 30-2 threshold exam using a size III stimulus from a 32-year-old woman with acute retrobulbar optic neuritis in the left eye. Her vision dropped to hand motions only during the acute episode. This field was performed seven weeks after the onset of symptoms when her acuity had improved to 20/30. There is generalized depression in addition to focal loss nasally. The nasal loss crosses the horizontal meridian. Also note the decreased foveal threshold. The field from the patient's asymptomatic right eye also shows inferonasal loss that crosses the horizontal meridian.

Figure 7-11 is a central 30-2 threshold exam from a 28-year-old woman who had an episode of optic neuritis 2 years earlier. Her visual acuity dropped to light perception during the acute episode and recovered to 20/60, where it has remained. She has subsequently developed other neurological abnormalities and has been diagnosed with multiple sclerosis. There is general reduction in sensitivity of the field with an area of focal depression centrally. Note the decreased foveal threshold.

Figure 7-11. Threshold exam of the right eye from a patient two years following an episode of optic neuritis.

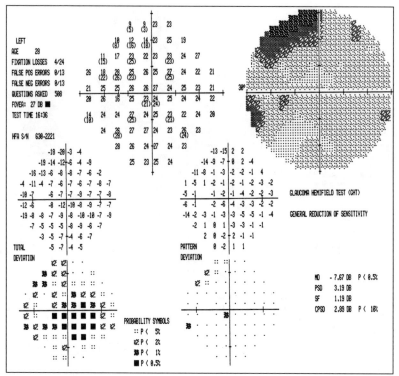

Figure 7-12 is a central 30-2 threshold test from a 38-year-old male with optic atrophy following optic neuritis and 20/200 vision in the eye. The reliability indices show a high number of fixation losses and a high false negative rate, suggestive of low patient reliability. In patients with loss of central fixation, small deviations in fixation are common and contribute to the high rate of fixation loss, a problem that is not unique to automated perimetry. Patients with moderately disturbed visual fields can have small shifts in fixation that move an area of non-seeing field onto an area in the projection bowl that the perimeter had previously established as seeing. Projection of a stimulus into this area during a false negative catchment trial will result in the stimulus not being seen and increase the false negative rate. The field also demonstrates a central scotoma with a foveal threshold of zero.

COMPRESSIVE OPTIC NEUROPATHY

Optic nerve compression can result from tumors, trauma, and orbital inflammatory disease. A patient with compressive optic neuropathy may present with proptosis, variable ocular motility deficits, decreased visual acuity, abnormal color vision, and an afferent pupillary defect. Usually the cause of the optic neuropathy will be determined from the patient's history and physical examination or by means of other testing, such as computed tomography. Automated perimetry is used in the setting of orbital disease to assist the clinician in detecting visual field loss, making interventional decisions, monitoring the course of the disease and effectiveness of therapy, and determining visual disability.

The central 30-2 threshold test from a 39-year-old man who was found to have an abnormality on confrontation fields in the left eye is shown in Figure 7-13. Examination revealed a visual acuity of 20/20 minus, mild color vision loss, an afferent pupillary defect, two millimeters of proptosis, and a swollen optic disc (Figure 7-14). Computed tomography of the orbits revealed an optic nerve meningioma with calcification of the nerve (Figure 7-15). The visual field reveals a ring-like scotoma, a generalized decrease in sensitivity, and decreased foveal threshold.

Figure 7-16 is a central 30-2 threshold test of the right eye of a 59-year-old woman with Graves' disease. She had noticed decreasing vision over several weeks and was found to have a right afferent pupillary defect and decreased color vision. Computed tomography revealed apical compression of the optic nerve by the extraocular muscles. The visual field reveals marked overall decreased sensitivity. The pattern deviation plot

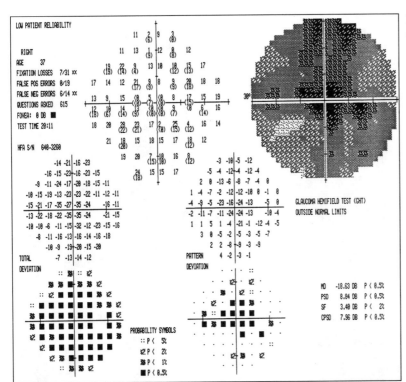

Figure 7-12. Threshold exam of the right eye from a patient with an optic atrophy.

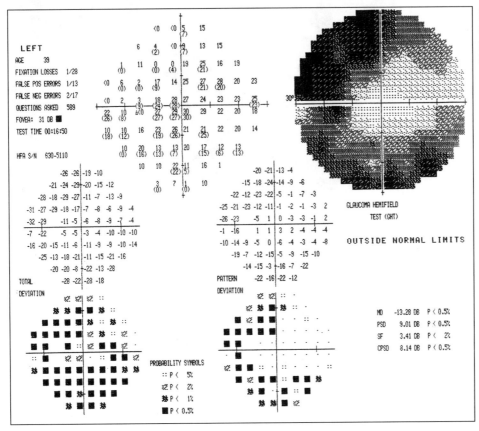

Figure 7-13. Threshold exam of the left eye from a patient with an optic nerve meningioma.

Figure 7-14. Left optic disc of the patient in Figure 7-13.

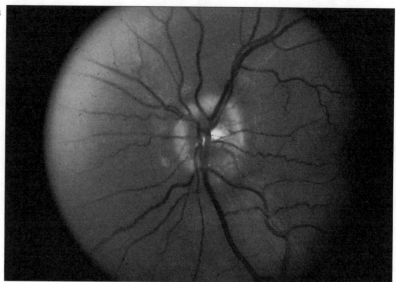

Figure 7-15. Computed axial tomography scan of the patient in Figure 7-13.

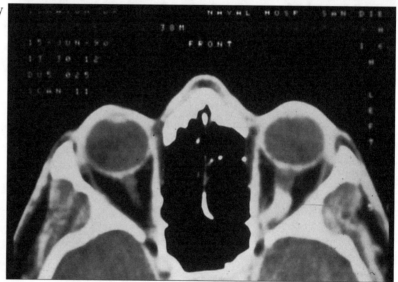

shows that the inferior hemifield has more loss than the superior. Figure 7-17 shows the field from the same eye following treatment.

Chiasmal Syndromes

The optic chiasm is the structure where the optic nerves come together and the axons originating in the nasal retina cross to join fibers from the opposite eye subserving the same side of visual space. These crossing fibers are more prone to injury than the fibers that do not cross. As a result, temporal field defects are the hallmark of chiasmal syndromes. Since the uncrossed fibers may be damaged as well, chiasmal field defects are not always limited to bitemporal hemianopias.

The optic chiasm may be affected by extrinsic (compressive) processes as well as by intrinsic (inflammatory or infiltrative) processes. Extrinsic causes, such as pituitary tumors, are more common than intrinsic causes, such as gliomas and chiasmal inflammation. The size, location, and extent of the lesion causing chiasmal syndrome will determine the visual field abnormality produced. Automated perimetry is useful in detecting visual field loss and monitoring the effectiveness of treatment in patients with chiasmal disease.

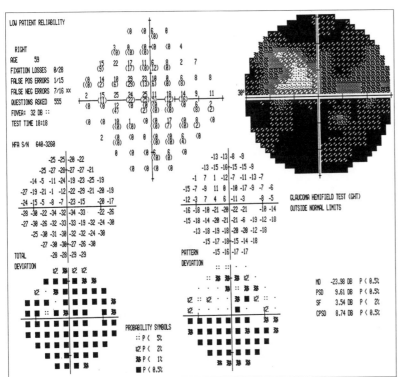

Figure 7-16. Threshold exam from a patient with optic neuropathy from Graves' disease.

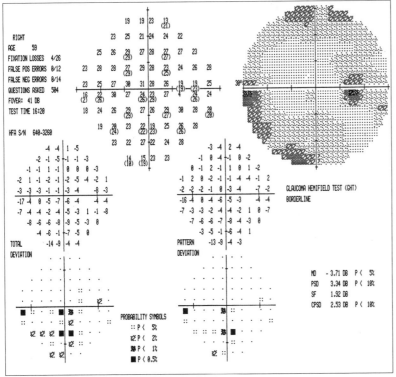

Figure 7-17. Threshold exam from the same patient as Figure 7-16, following therapy.

Figure 7-18, left. Visual field series from the left eye of a patient with a pituitary tumor showing development of a superior bitemporal hemianopia in a patient. The visual field defect resolved following surgical removal of the tumor.

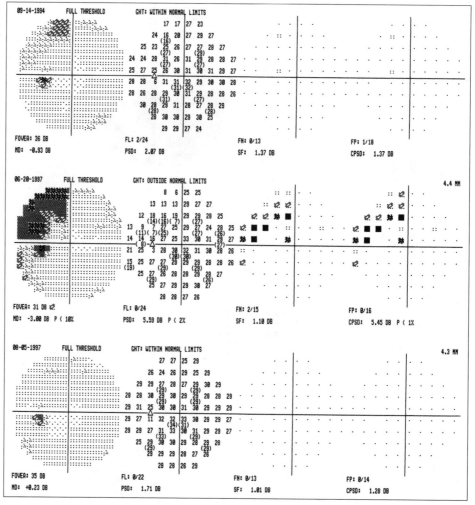

Figure 7-18 shows a bitemporal hemianopia developing in a patient with a pituitary tumor. As can be seen in the third field in the series, the defect resolved following removal of the tumor. The central 30-2 threshold test from the left and right eyes of a 51-year-old visually asymptomatic man who was undergoing an endocrine evaluation for a low thyroid-stimulating hormone level in the presence of low thyroxine level is shown in Figure 7-19. Neuro-imaging of the chiasm was obtained, revealing a macroadenoma of the pituitary. The field shows an obvious defect in the left eye with only a small superior temporal defect in the right eye. Following trans-sphenoidal surgery, the field defects are markedly improved (Figure 7-20).

Figure 7-21 shows central 30-2 threshold test of the left and right eyes of a 33-year-old man who presented with decreased visual acuity. His visual acuity was 20/25 in the right eye and 20/100 in the left with a left-sided afferent pupillary defect and loss of color vision. The pattern of field loss is that of a junctional scotoma (ie, loss of central vision in one eye and a temporal defect in the other). This type of visual field defect localizes the responsible lesion to the place where the optic nerve on the side with the greater loss joins the chiasm. Neuro-imaging revealed a large sellar mass that was found to be a nonsecreting pituitary adenoma. Following surgery, the patient's visual acuity improved, but he was left with an incongruous right hemianopia and a left inferior nerve fiber bundle defect (Figure 7-22).

Figure 7-23 is a central 30-2 threshold test of both eyes in a 45-year-old man who suffered a skull fracture in a motorcycle accident 15 years earlier. It shows a classical bitemporal field defect.

Figure 7-24 is a central 30-2 threshold test of both eyes of a 49-year-old man who noted a nine-day history of progressive of visual disturbance in both eyes. He had normal visual acuity, normal color vision, and no afferent defect. The visual fields show inferior paracentral temporal defects in each eye. Magnetic resonance imaging of the chiasm revealed an enlarged chiasm that enhanced with gadolinium. He received pulse

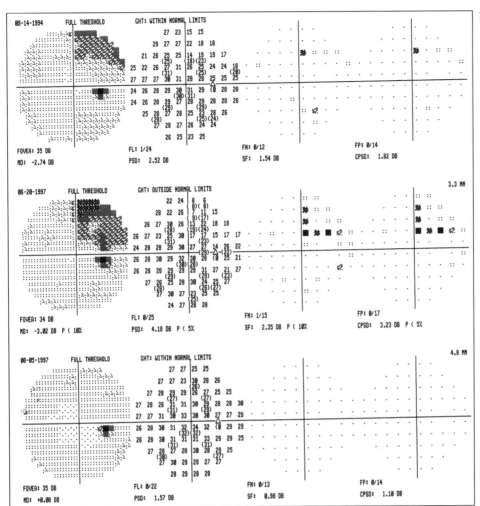

Figure 7-18, right.

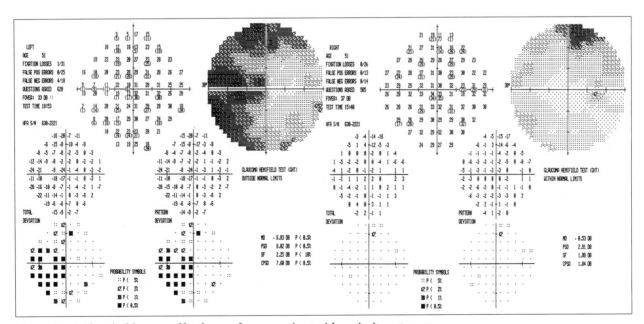

Figure 7-19. Threshold exam of both eyes from a patient with a pituitary tumor.

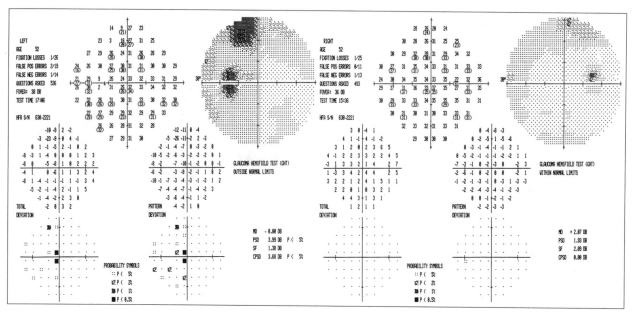

Figure 7-20. Threshold exam from the same patient as in Figure 7-19, following trans-sphenoidal pituitary surgery.

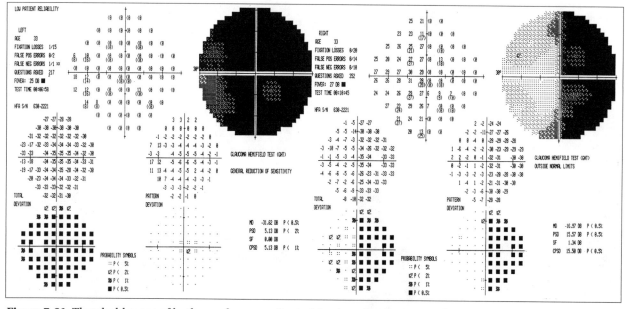

Figure 7-21. Threshold exam of both eyes from a patient with a junctional scotoma from a pituitary tumor.

intravenous corticosteroids. His inflammatory chiasmal syndrome improved but did not completely resolve. The patient continues to exhibit Uthoff's phenomenon with worsening of his bitemporal field defects during periods of exercise and in hot showers.

Retrochiasmal Lesions

Following the hemidecussation at the optic chiasm, visual pathway axons on the right side carry information about visual space to the left and axons on the left carry information about visual space to the right. Central nervous system lesions posterior to the chiasm causing visual field defects therefore cause homonymous hemianopias. For incomplete homonymous hemianopias, the more congruous the field defect, the more posterior the lesion. Figure 7-22, previously discussed, is an example of a noncongruous homonymous hemi-

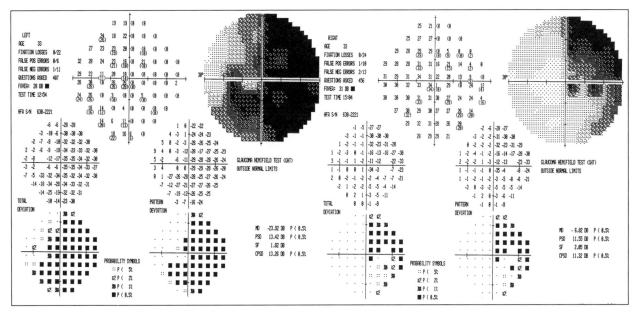

Figure 7-22. Threshold exam from the same patient as in Figure 7-21, following surgery.

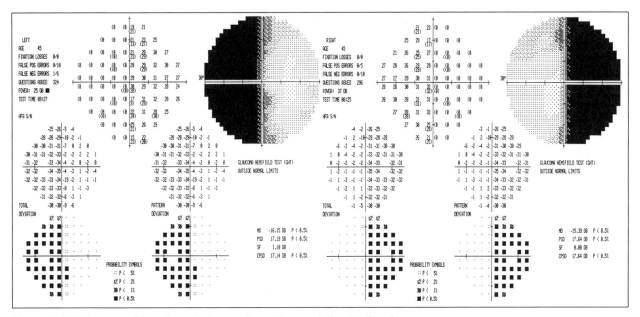

Figure 7-23. Bitemporal hemianopia in a patient 15 years following head trauma.

anopia. Complete hemianopias, on the other hand, only establish a lesion as retrochiasmal. Tumor, stroke, inflammatory disease, congenital anomalies, and trauma can all be causes of retrochiasmal field defects.

A 66-year-old man complained of a left-sided visual disturbance and left-sided clumsiness for 2 1/2 weeks. His visual fields are shown in Figure 7-25. Neuro-imaging revealed a right occipitoparietal mass that was thought to be metastatic in nature. The fields show a complete left homonymous hemianopia. Additional examples of homonymous defects can be seen in Figures 7-26 through 7-29. Figure 7-26 shows an example of bilateral occipital lobe infarctions. Figures 7-27a through 7-27d show a change in the pattern of loss in a glaucoma patient with the development of a homonymous defect. Investigation revealed metastatic lung cancer. Figure 7-28 is a central 30-2 threshold test of the left and right eyes of a 25-year-old man with a history of migraine who was found to have trouble with confrontation fields to the left side. The fields show a congruous left superior quadrantic defect. A computed tomography scan revealed encephalomalacia of a portion

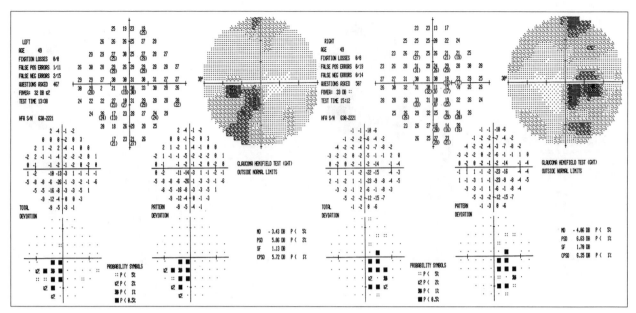

Figure 7-24. Threshold exam of both eyes from a patient with a chiasmal inflammatory syndrome.

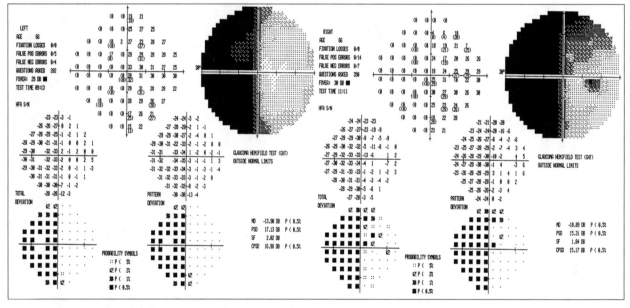

Figure 7-25. Complete left homonymous hemianopia from a parieto-occipital tumor.

of the right occipital lobe. Figure 7-29 is a similar set of fields in a 73-year-old male who had a right occipital lobe infarct.

Nonorganic Visual Loss

Patients with nonorganic visual loss can be difficult. Visual field testing has long been a mainstay in establishing the diagnosis of nonorganic visual loss. Nonexpanding and spiral fields are nonphysiologic in nature and are commonly found in such patients. The Humphrey perimeter does not permit these types of abnormalities to be readily measured; tangent screen testing and Goldmann perimetry are both useful in establishing the nonphysiologic nature of some visual field abnormalities. Nonetheless, there are some find-

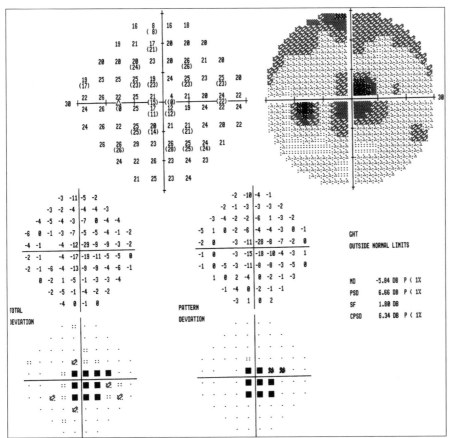

Figure 7-26, left. At first glance this patient appears to have bilateral central scotomata. However, she had good visual acuity in each eye and a normal appearing retina OU. This visual field from the left eye are consistent with bilateral occipital lobe infarctions.

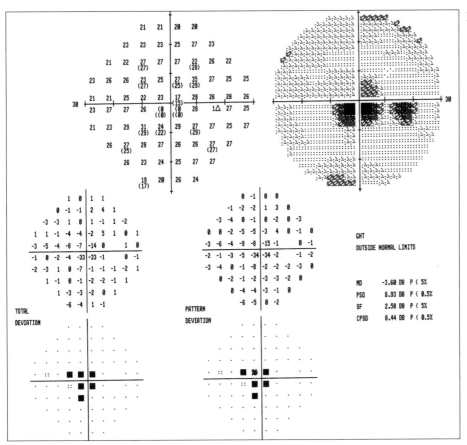

Figure 7-26, right.

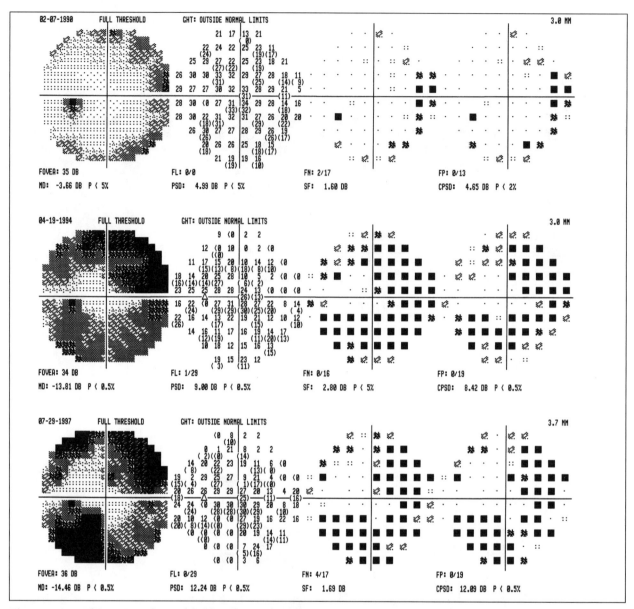

Figure 7-27a. This series of visual fields is from the left eye of a patient with open-angle glaucoma and shows development of glaucomatous visual field loss between the first and second exams. It may appear that the field has worsened in the third exam, but closer inspection of the inferior quadrant of the left eye shows the new loss to be hemianopic and not consistent with progression of glaucoma.

ings with automated perimetry that can be very suggestive of nonorganic loss. Recognition of these findings can assist the clinician with these difficult and time-consuming patients.

Irreproducibility of a pattern of loss with automated perimetry is one clue to nonphysiologic visual field loss. Patients suspected of malingering will sometimes reveal vastly different patterns of field loss on repeat testing. High short-term fluctuations and false negatives may also be clues. When a patient has visual field loss that does not "fit" with the remainder of his examination, the clinician should look for these signs of irreproducibility by repeating the examination. One pattern of field loss that is very common in nonphysiologic visual loss is a severely constricted field with relatively normal central and foveal threshold values in the presence of decreased visual acuity. Figure 7-30 is an example of such fields.

The differential diagnosis of "tunnel" fields and their distinguishing characteristics can be found in Table 7-1.

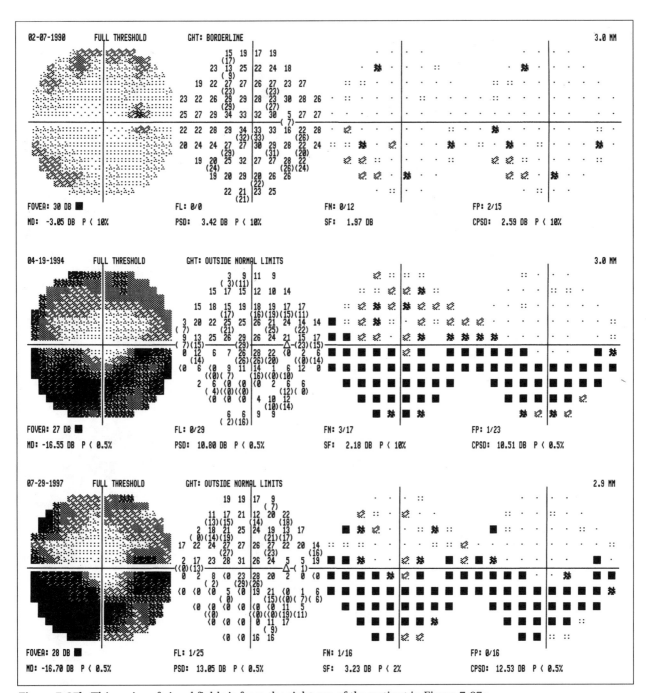

Figure 7-27b. This series of visual fields is from the right eye of the patient in Figure 7-27a.

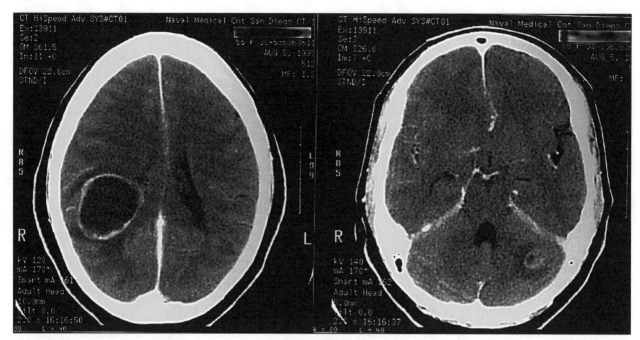

Figure 7-27c. The patient in Figures 7-27 a and b underwent neuro-imaging and was found to have a large mass in the right parietal lobe, responsible for the new hemianopic defect. However, there was a smaller mass in the left side of the cerebellum, indicative of metastatic disease.

Figure 7-27d. The patient in Figures 7-27a, b, and c underwent a chest x-ray that revealed a large mass, found to be an oat cell carcinoma.

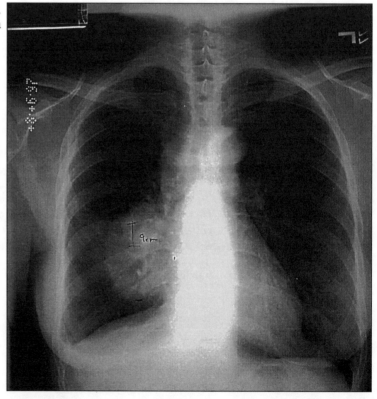

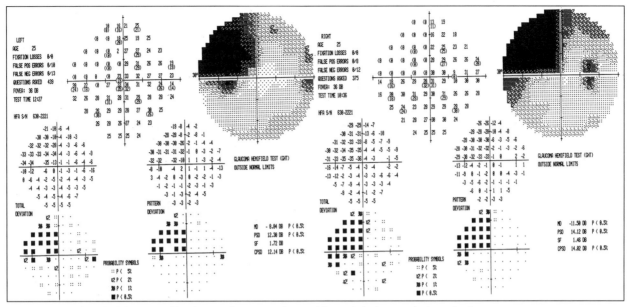

Figure 7-28. Threshold exam of both eyes from a patient with occipital encephalomalacia.

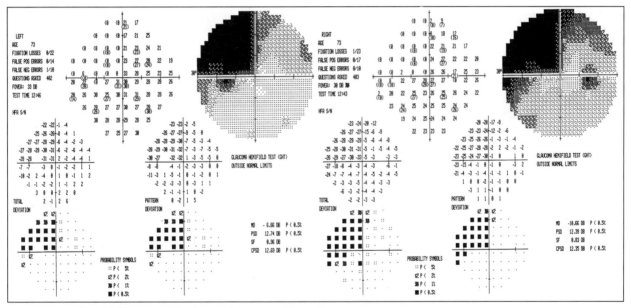

Figure 7-29. Threshold exam of both eyes from a stroke patient.

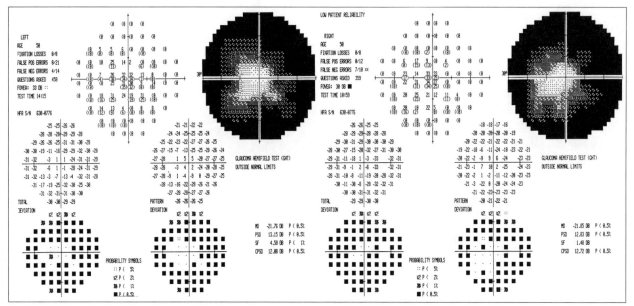

Figure 7-30. Threshold exam of both eyes of a patient with nonphysiologic visual loss.

Table 7-1

DIFFERENTIAL DIAGNOSIS FOR "TUNNEL" VISUAL FIELDS

Cause	Clues
Glaucoma	IOP, advanced cupping
Retinitis pigmentosa	Retinal exam, electroretinography
Optic neuropathy	Fundus exam, afferent defect (if unilateral)
Nonphysiologic	Inter- and intratest variability, tangent screen (spiral, nonexpanding)

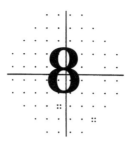

Visual Field Defects from Miscellaneous Conditions

Introduction

The vast majority of visual field testing is carried out to detect disease known to cause visual field damage. Patients found to have elevated intraocular pressure who are thought to be at risk for having or developing glaucoma will undergo visual field testing for loss consistent with the diagnosis of glaucoma or to establish a "baseline" visual field against which future tests can be measured for change. Visual field changes in glaucoma are discussed in Chapter 6. Patients with neurological conditions often undergo visual field testing to help the clinician pinpoint the location of lesions in the visual pathways. Visual field defects related to neuro-ophthalmology and neurologic conditions are discussed in Chapter 7. The diagnosis of conditions related to other parts of the eye usually does not involve visual field testing, because most of those conditions are not expected to involve the visual fields or the diagnosis can be made by either examination alone or some other diagnostic modality.

This chapter presents, in atlas format, a collection of visual fields that were administered for reasons other than glaucoma and neuro-ophthalmology. It is not intended to be a complete collection of visual fields from every possible ophthalmic disorder, but representative of most of the entities encountered in clinical practice. Some of the defects are of interest because they closely resemble those found in glaucoma and are presented because they are part of the "differential diagnosis" of glaucomatous visual field loss. Many conditions can cause "cupping," and such patients often undergo visual field testing to see if it is from glaucoma. Table 8-1 lists some of the nonglaucoma conditions thought to be causes for cupping.

Some of the fields presented in this chapter were administered as part of the "shotgun" approach to a patient with an unknown condition (ie, "we don't know what this is, let's get a visual field and see if that helps"). Some patients whose diagnoses were known underwent visual field testing to quantitate the extent of their loss for counseling purposes, disability ratings, or as a baseline for follow-up. Other fields presented came about because the patient had a complaint of visual field loss or some other visual defect and the cause was not apparent upon examination, while others are of interest because they represent real damage that does not fit visual field loss patterns previously presented in this book. Finally, some of these cases are examples in which the diagnosis was made upon clinical examination, and the provider thought the visual field would be "interesting."

Table 8-1

Nonglaucomatous Causes for Cupping

General Category	Examples	Differential Test(s)
Compressive lesions	Meningioma, aneurysm, intracranial tumor	Exophthalmometry, motility, neuro-imaging (CT, MRI)
Ischemia	Ischemic optic neuropathy, temporal arteritis	CBC (anemia), erythrocyte sedimentation rate, temporal artery biopsy
Post-inflammatory	Optic neuritis, multiple sclerosis, syphilis	History, serology (VDRL, FTA-ABS, MHATP), MRI
Trauma	Traumatic optic neuropathy	History
Congenital anomalies	Colobomata, optic nerve pits, drusen	Clinical appearance
Toxic optic neuropathies	Ethambutol	History
Optic atrophy	Idiopathic, familial dominant	Family history

Structural Defects of the Optic Nerve

CONGENITAL DEFECTS

Enlargement of the Blind Spot

Since there are no photoreceptors on the surface of the optic nerve head, the area of the visual field containing the nerve head (15° temporally, straddling the horizontal midline) will appear as a "hole" in the visual field, known as the physiologic blind spot. A larger than normal blind spot has been thought to be of clinical significance. Rather than an indicator of acquired disease, enlargement of the blind spot usually represents a congenital variation of the structure of the optic nerve or some other variation of normal. Figure 8-1(disc) is the disc photograph from such a patient with a congenitally aberrant optic nerve. There is a large pigmented temporal crescent, indicating that the retina does not quite reach to the margin of the disc and the underlying choroid is exposed. Figure 8-1 (field) is the visual field from this eye. The blind spot shows very mild enlargement corresponding to the pigmented crescent. Another example is shown in Figure 8-2 (disc and field). There is a large scleral crescent, probably with exposed sclera visible, and multiple depressed points surrounding the center of the blind spot. The area of the probable blind spot has been circled in Figure 8-2F.

Colobomata

Failure of the fetal fissure to close results in a defect in the inferotemporal aspect of the optic nerve, known as a coloboma. Occasionally, structural defects will occur in the superior pole of the disc, resulting in inferior visual field defects. Two such examples are shown in Figures 8-3 and 8-4. The disc photographs and visual fields are shown from both eyes of these two patients. The remarkable aspects of these two cases are the symmetrical malformations of the superior poles of both optic nerves in each case and the similar inferior visual field defects in both eyes of both cases. If you look closely at Figure 8-4 (disc), right and left, you can see the absence of nerve fibers at the superior pole of both nerves.

Optic Pit

A structural defect in the temporal aspect of the optic nerve head may occur with the appearance of a localized excavation. One such typical optic pit is shown in Figure 8-5 (disc), and the corresponding visual

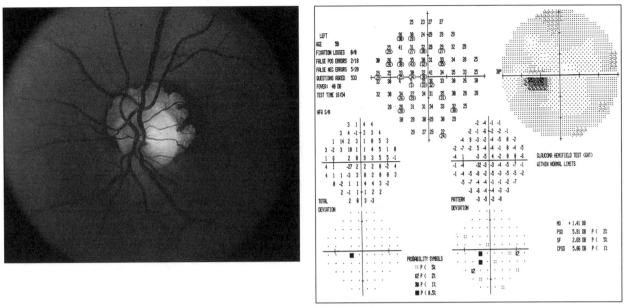

Figure 8-1. Disc photograph and visual field from a patient with a congenitally aberrant optic nerve, showing a scleral crescent and slight enlargement of the blind spot.

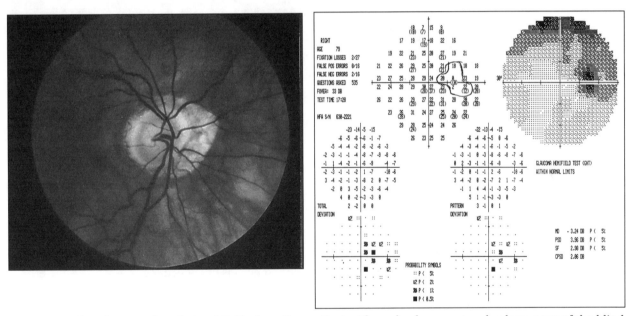

Figure 8-2. Disc photograph and visual field of another patient with a scleral crescent and enlargement of the blind spot.

field is shown in Figure 8-5 (field). The visual field defect is a typical nerve fiber bundle defect and could easily be confused with a glaucomatous defect.

Acquired Defects

Optic Nerve Drusen

Optic nerve drusen have been discussed in Chapter 7. Another example is given in Figure 8-6. This patient was followed as a glaucoma suspect because of the characteristic inferior nasal step resembling the

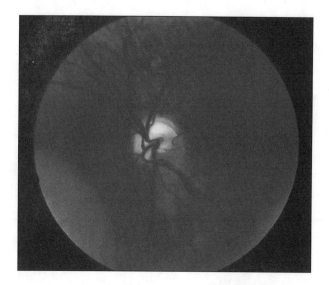
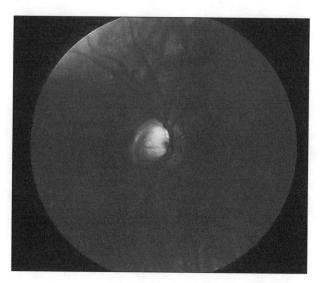

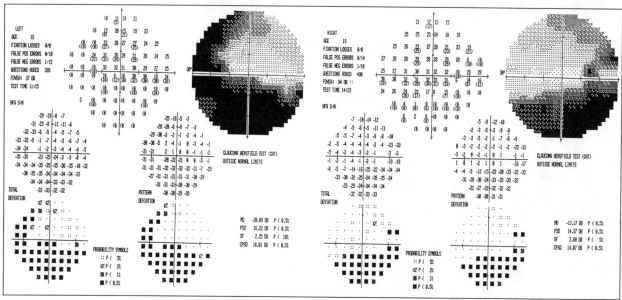

Figure 8-3. Disc photographs and visual fields from a patient with an atypical coloboma of the optic nerve head.

defect seen in glaucoma. These visual field defects are acquired because they occur as buried drusen "erupt" to the surface of the nerve, starting in childhood.

Optic Atrophy

The disc photographs of a patient with mild sectoral optic atrophy are shown in Figure 8-7 (disc), right and left. The is mild pallor without cupping on the temporal side of the nerve, right eye worse than the left. The etiology of the atrophy in this patient is not known. The patient underwent a screening visual field using the 120-point full field screen with the three-zone strategy. The results are shown in Figure 8-7 (field). The loss pattern is suggestive of nerve fiber bundle defects, but the magnitude of the defects is not known because only the screening test was performed.

Melanocytoma

The patient whose disc photograph is shown in Figure 8-8 (disc) has a small, benign pigmented tumor on his optic nerve head, known as a melanocytoma. The corresponding visual field (Figure 8-8 [field]), a 24-2, shows defects similar to those seen in patients with glaucoma.

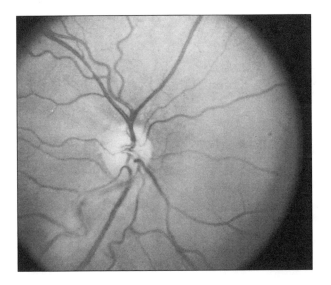
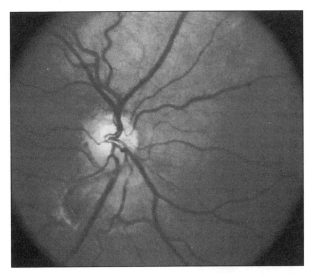

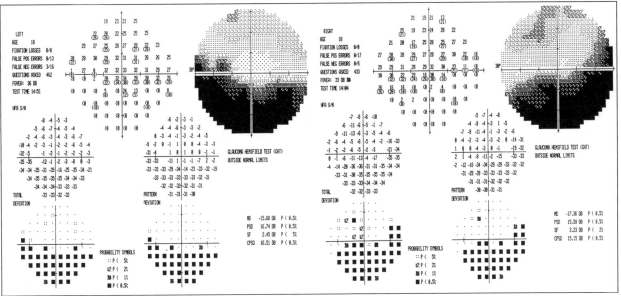

Figure 8-4. Another example of disc photographs and visual fields of a patient with a congenitally malformed optic nerve.

"It Just Got in My Way"

CATARACT

The various causes for diffuse loss of sensitivity have been described in Chapter 5. Figure 8-9 is another example of a patient with a cataract. This patient had mild ocular hypertension and was followed with visual fields. The first field in the overview analysis in Figure 8-9 demonstrates mild diffuse loss and a "graytone construction artifact" suggestive of focal superior loss. The cataract was removed one month after this visual field was done, and the overview analysis demonstrates that no loss is present and the field has remained stable for four years.

PTOSIS

The eyelid artifact has been described in Chapter 5. However, sometimes the upper lid really does get in the way. The first visual field in the overview analysis shown in Figure 8-10 demonstrates a significant loss

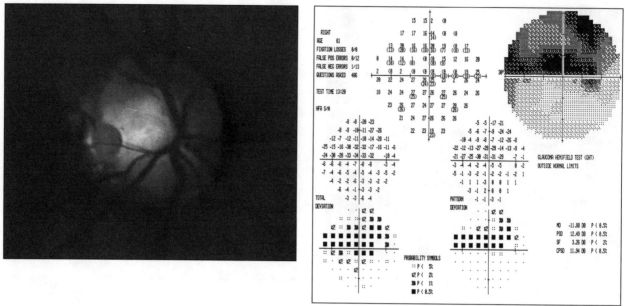

Figure 8-5. Disc photo and visual field from a patient with a congenital optic pit.

Figure 8-6. Visual field from a patient with optic nerve head drusen.

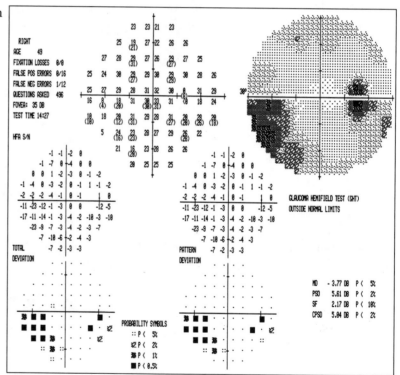

of the superior visual field attributed to ptosis and marked dermatochalasis with hooding of the upper lid. The visual field was repeated with the eyelid taped open, and the result is shown as the second visual field in the overview.

Trauma

Manifestations of ocular trauma are varied and the results of visual field testing will, of course, depend on the location and extent of the injury. The patient whose visual field is shown in Figure 8-11 complained

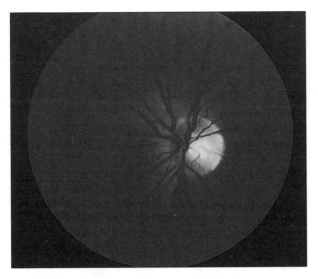
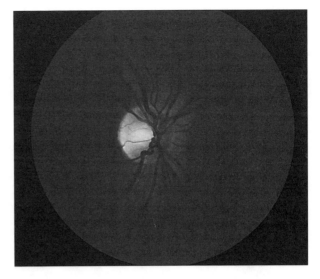

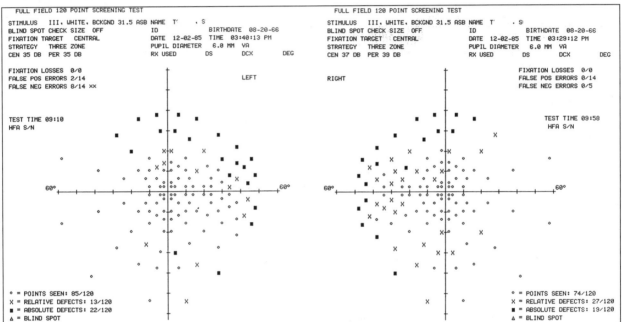

Figure 8-7. Optic nerve photographs and visual fields of a patient with mild optic atrophy of unknown etiology.

of a "spot" in front of his right eye. The 30-2 test revealed one disturbed paracentral point in the superotemporal quadrant (26 dB sensitivity, circled). A 10-2 test was done to further explore this disturbed area of the visual field (Figure 8-12). Note that this paracentral defect does not respect the horizontal midline and must therefore be of retinal origin. The patient's history was such that he may have been accidentally exposed to some sort of laser, and it is suspected that this is a laser injury. There was a subtle retinal pigment epithelial defect present in the fundus, which is compatible with this sort of injury.

Blunt trauma can cause significant intraocular injury, as is the case of the patient whose fundus photo is shown in Figure 8-13 (disc). The visual field defects corresponding to the inferonasal choroidal rupture and macular scarring are shown in Figure 8-13 (field). Since the paracentral defect and temporal wedge defect respect the horizontal, these could be mistaken for disc-based defects.

The patient shown in Figure 8-14 suffered closed head trauma after being thrown from a motorcycle. There were no direct injuries identified to her eyes or any part of her visual pathway. She was, however, in shock for a significant amount of time and appeared to have sustained an injury to her optic nerves, known as *shock optic neuropathy*. The optic nerves appear cupped with central pallor (Figure 8-14 [disc]). The visu-

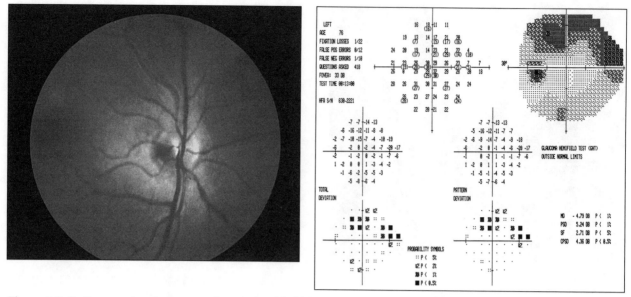

Figure 8-8. Optic nerve head photograph and visual field from a patient with a melanocytoma.

al fields (Figure 8-14 [field], right and left) show nerve fiber bundle loss, right eye much worse than left. The top of the figure for each eye is a 120-point screen with the three-zone strategy, and the bottom is a 30-2 performed approximately two months later. The left eye shows minimal loss, and the defect shown may be a rim artifact. The right eye, however, shows an altitudinal hemianopia compatible with significant optic nerve injury.

Post-Inflammatory Changes

Loss of vision following inflammatory disease in the visual system is related to destruction of tissue from the inflammatory process and replacement of tissue with scars. The visual field shown in Figure 8-15 (field) shows a typical inferior arcuate scotoma. The etiology of this defect is a retinal scar due to toxoplasmosis. The fundus photograph is Figure 8-15 (disc). Figure 8-16 (field) is an end-stage visual field. The cause of this extensive visual field loss was optic neuritis due to syphilis. The disc photo, demonstrating marked pallor, cupping, and atrophy, is shown in Figure 8-16 (disc).

Presumed Vascular or Circulatory Problems

The patient whose visual fields are shown in Figure 8-17 was under treatment for low-tension glaucoma. Each eye shows a disc-based superior nerve fiber bundle defect, and the optic nerves are missing rim tissue at their inferior poles. These defects developed after the patient underwent uncomplicated coronary artery bypass grafting and probably represent another form of shock optic neuropathy. His ocular medications were discontinued and his intraocular pressure remained in the low to mid teens with no change in these visual fields over time.

Vascular accidents would be expected to affect the visual field if a portion of the visual pathway was involved. Field defects from cerebral vascular accidents were discussed in Chapter 7. The patient shown in Figure 8-18 had an occlusion of a cilioretinal artery. The resulting defect is therefore retinal based, rather than optic nerve based. It does, however, resemble the disc-based defects seen in glaucoma or mimicking syndromes (Figure 8-15) and would be difficult to diagnose correctly without the proper history. The defect on the total deviation plot straddles the midline, as would be expected for a visual field defect due to a retinal lesion. There is also mild reduction in foveal threshold, which is compatible with this artery occlusion.

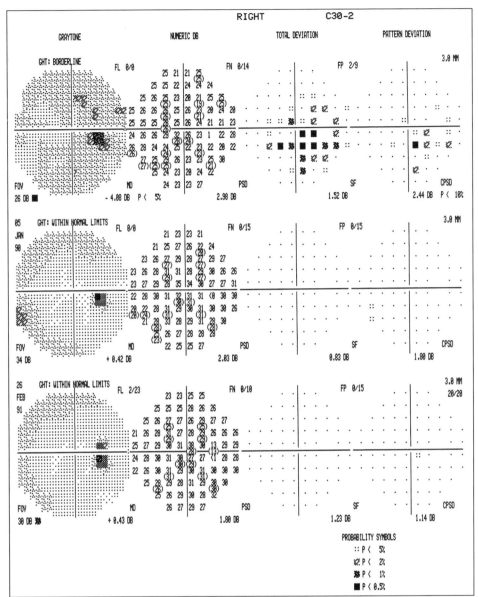

Figure 8-9. Visual field change over time in a patient with cataract, before and after removal.

Figure 8-19 is from a patient with background diabetic retinopathy who underwent focal argon laser photocoagulation. The field shows a reduction in foveal threshold (20 dB [decibels]), central loss, diffuse loss, and some constriction. The central loss is attributable to diabetic macular edema.

The next two patients have in common a history of hypertensive crisis. The patient shown in Figure 8-20 complained of loss of vision in the center while retaining good visual acuity. The fields show bilateral central scotomata with relatively good foveal thresholds. The macular threshold program was performed to zoom in on the center of the field (Figure 8-21). The etiology of these defects is presumed to be an occipital lobe infarction.

Hypertensive crisis can occur as a complication of pregnancy, as experienced by the patient whose visual fields are shown in Figures 8-22, 8-23, and 8-24. She was not seen by an ophthalmologist during the acute episode, but rather weeks after the crisis. She complained of loss of peripheral vision from her left eye only, involving the lower left portion of her vision. The visual field loss detected on the 30-2 was only at the edge and could have been artifactual. Because of her insistence on the extent of the loss, a peripheral 30/60 threshold test was performed. Thus, threshold testing out to 60° was performed, and the threshold values are displayed in Figure 8-22. Note the significant loss of sensitivity in the inferior temporal quadrant as manifested by the "quad total" (compare to the other three quadrants). The defect depth printout is Figure 8-23, and the

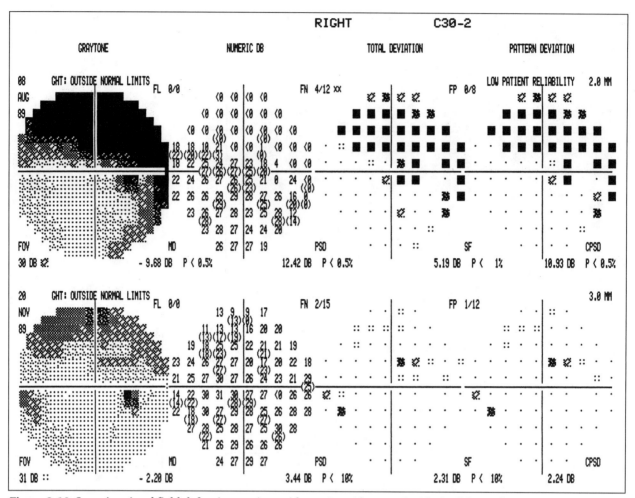

Figure 8-10. Superior visual field defect in a patient with ptosis, without and with the lid taped open.

graytone printout is Figure 8-24. The etiology of this defect is hard to pinpoint, but it is unilateral and therefore anterior to the chiasm (ie, optic nerve based). It most likely represents a segmental ischemic optic neuropathy.

Retinal Disease

Except as noted in the introduction to this chapter, the majority of patients with retinal disease do not require visual field testing since most of their disease is visible ophthalmoscopically. The patient illustrated in Figure 8-25 is a 93-year-old with age-related macular degeneration. His foveal thresholds are reduced, right greater than left, and he has central depressions, right greater than left.

The visual field shown in Figure 8-26 is that of a patient with a macular hole. Even though the field was tested with the central fixation target, the defect and blind spot appear to be shifted down because the patient is using his peripheral vision to fixate. His eye was thus rotated during the test.

Patients with retinal detachments rarely require field testing. The patient whose visual field is shown in Figure 8-27 underwent retinal detachment repair and complained of visual field loss. Although initially thought by a non-ophthalmologist to have redetached, clinical examination did not bear this out. A visual field was administered because of his complaints. This loss pattern should never be confused with disc-based or neurological field loss because it does not respect either meridian. This patient did not have an acute process.

Figure 8-28 shows visual field changes (a) and the retinal appearance (b) in a patient with neuroretinitis from catscratch disease.

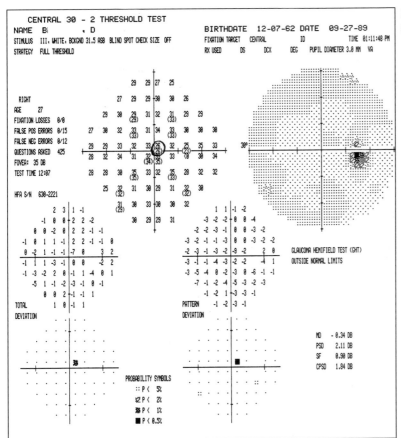

Figure 8-11. Paracentral defect from a presumed laser injury.

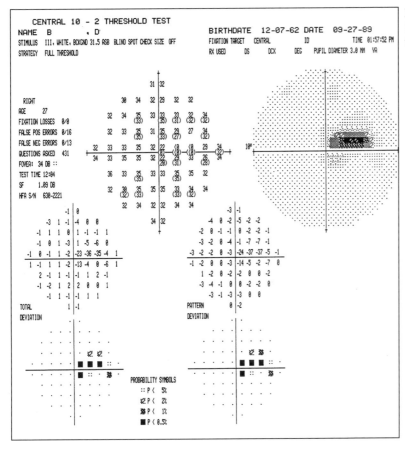

Figure 8-12. Same patient as in Figure 8-11, with a close-up of the defect found on the 30-2 test.

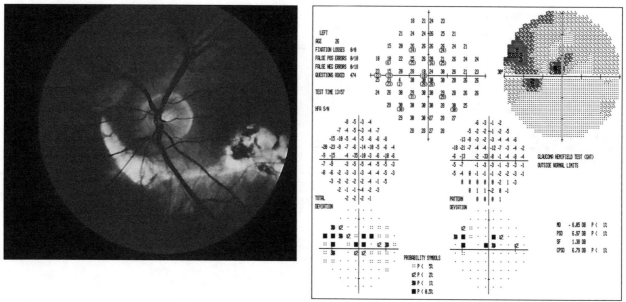

Figure 8-13. Fundus photograph and visual field from an eye status post-blunt trauma with a choroidal rupture and macular scarring.

Patients with retinal dystrophies often require visual field testing, either to document the extent of their loss for disability purposes or for diagnostic purposes when the diagnosis is not ophthalmoscopically obvious. Figures 8-29 and 8-30 are from patients with retinal dystrophies. The patient illustrated in Figure 8-29 has a rod-cone dystrophy. He noted difficulty with night vision tasks. The diagnosis was made electrophysiologically. Both eyes demonstrate diffuse depression, and the left eye has a classic "ring" scotoma. The patient in Figure 8-30 has retinitis pigmentosa with severe field loss, right much worse than left. Note the right eye required a stimulus V. The field was totally black to stimulus III. Another example is given in Figure 8-31. Retinitis pigmentosa is one of the "night blindness" disorders characterized by abnormal retinal pigmentation, loss of peripheral visual field, difficulty adapting to and seeing in the dark, "waxy" pallor of the optic nerve, arteriolar narrowing, cataract formation, and macular changes. The electroretinogram (ERG) shows a typical extinction pattern. Figures 8-31a through 8-31d shows the typical visual field constriction and ERG extinction pattern of retinitis pigmentosa.

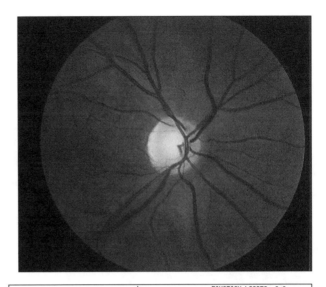

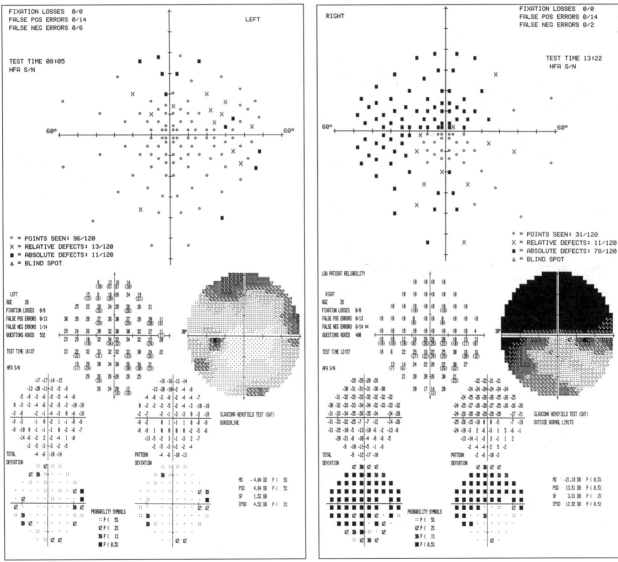

Figure 8-14. Disc photograph from the right eye and visual fields from both eyes of a patient who sustained presumed shock optic neuropathy following closed head trauma.

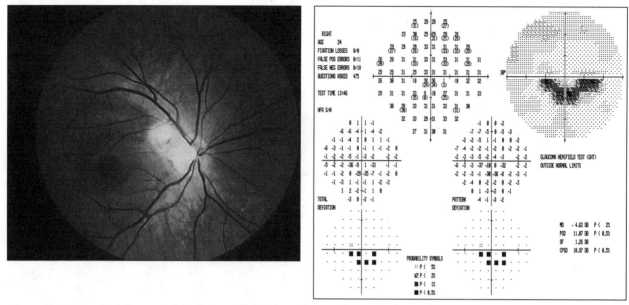

Figure 8-15. Fundus photograph and visual field of a patient with a retinal scar due to ocular toxoplasmosis.

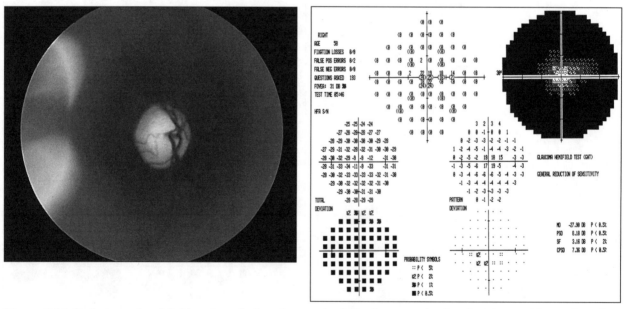

Figure 8-16. End-stage visual field and marked optic atrophy following an episode of optic neuritis attributed to syphilis.

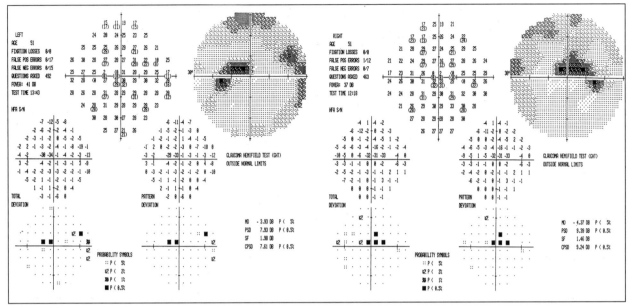

Figure 8-17. Bilateral nerve fiber bundle defects developing following open heart surgery, presumably due to shock.

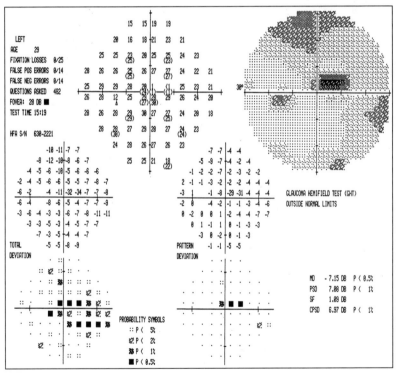

Figure 8-18. Visual field defect from occlusion of a cilioretinal artery.

Figure 8-19. Visual field defects in a patient with background diabetic retinopathy.

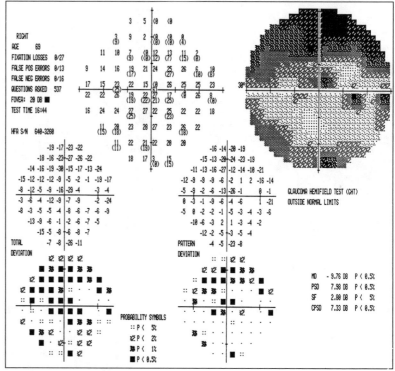

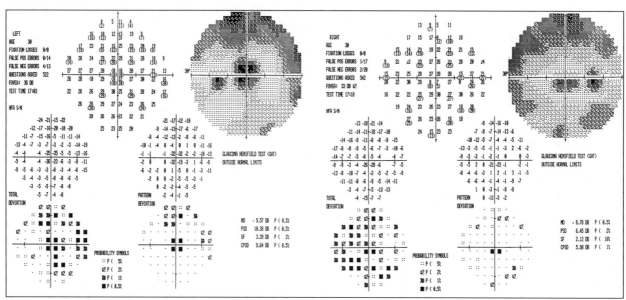

Figure 8-20. Central visual field loss following a hypertensive crisis.

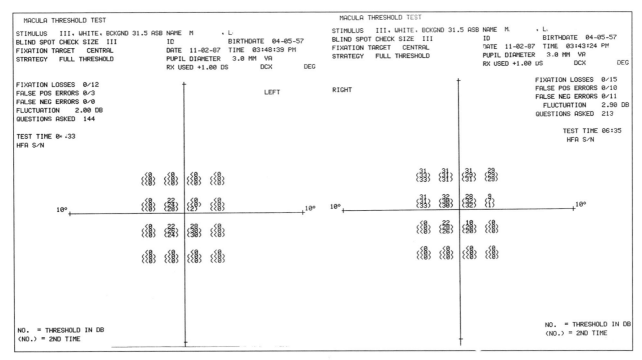

Figure 8-21. Macular threshold program from the patient shown in Figure 8-20.

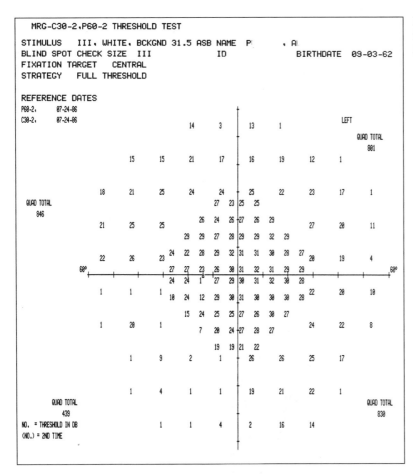

Figure 8-22. Peripheral visual field loss following a hypertensive crisis, merged 30-2 and peripheral 30/60, value table.

Figure 8-23. Peripheral visual field loss following a hypertensive crisis, merged 30-2 and peripheral 30/60, defect depth printout.

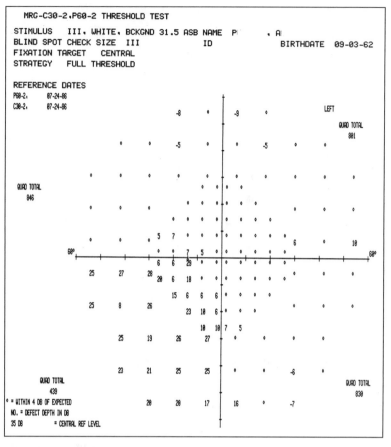

Figure 8-24. Peripheral visual field loss following a hypertensive crisis, merged 30-2 and peripheral 30/60, graytone printout.

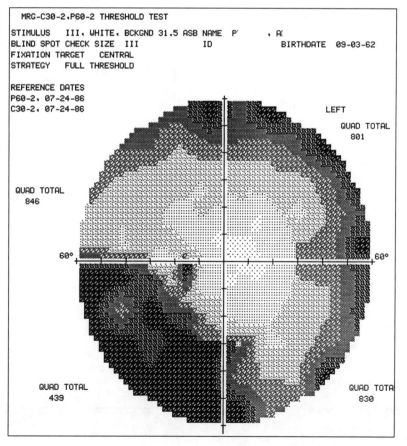

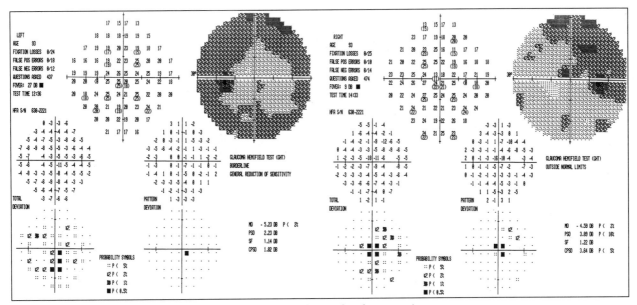

Figure 8-25. Visual fields from a patient with age-related macular degeneration.

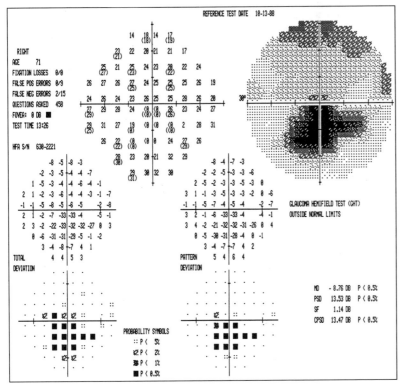

Figure 8-26. Central visual field defect due to a macular hole.

Figure 8-27. Visual field defects in a patient with a retinal detachment.

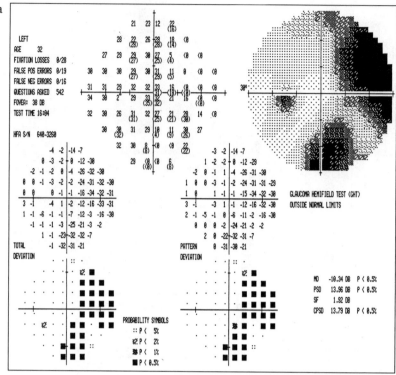

Figure 8-28a. An example of a cecocentral scotoma in a patient with neuroretinitis determined to be from cat-scratch disease.

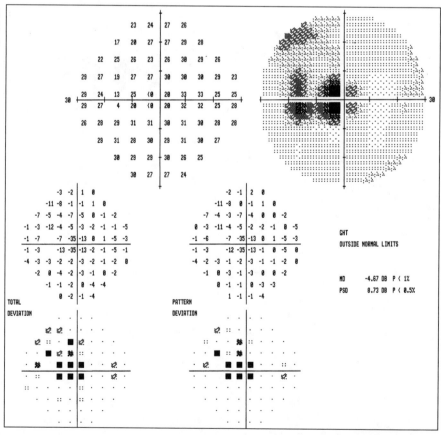

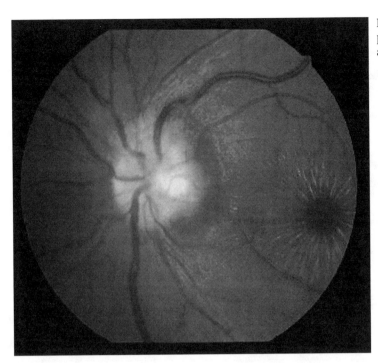

Figure 8-28b. The fundus photograph of the patient in Figure 8-28a shows optic disc edema and a macular star.

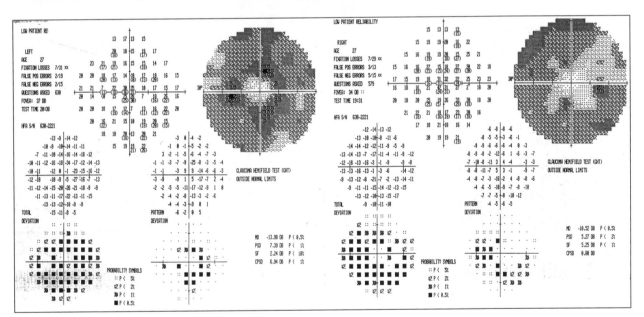

Figure 8-29. Visual field loss due to rod-cone dystrophy.

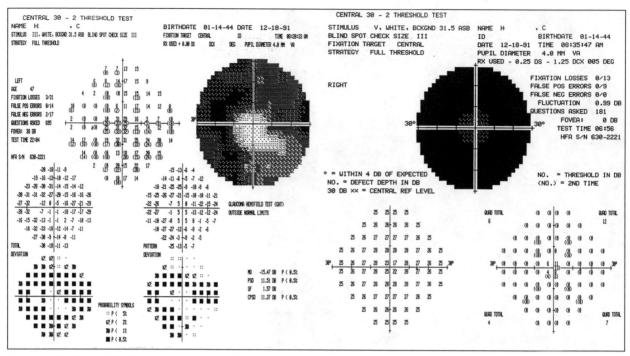

Figure 8-30. Visual field loss in a patient with retinitis pigmentosa.

Figure 8-31a. Constricted visual field of the left eye of a patient with retinitis pigmentosa.

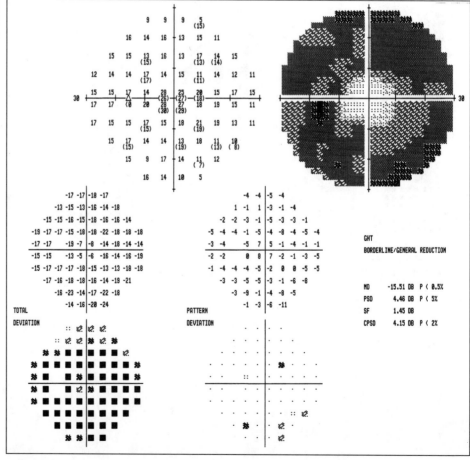

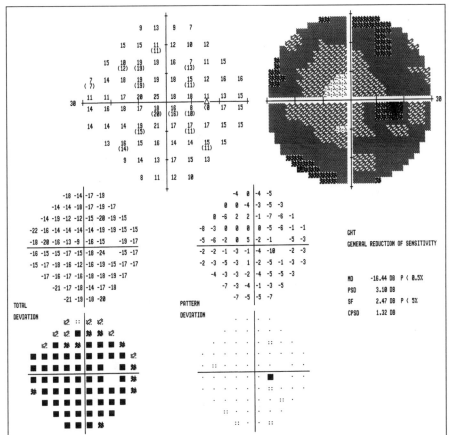

Figure 8-31b. Constricted visual field of the right eye of the patient in Figure 8-31a with retinitis pigmentosa. The electroretinogram (Figure 8-31c) shows extinction in both eyes.

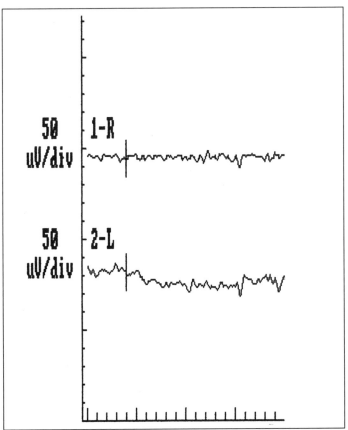

Figure 8-31c. The electroretinogram of the patient in Figures 8-31a and 8-31b shows extinction in both eyes.

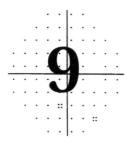

Latest Innovations for the Humphrey Field Analyzer

Introduction

Since the introduction of the Humphrey Field Analyzer, Humphrey Instruments has been attentive to the needs and desires of its customers. The operating software for the instrument has been updated on a regular basis, incorporating changes that have made the perimeter more user friendly and kinder to the patient. STATPAC and STATPAC 2 are software options that add age-corrected normal comparisons to threshold testing, thus incorporating into the Humphrey perimeter analysis techniques desired by the machine users. FASTPAC was introduced in an attempt to meet the desire to decrease testing time for threshold tests. This chapter discusses other available options for the Humphrey Field Analyzer and includes items on the horizon.

Short-Wavelength Automated Perimetry

Pamela A. Sample, PhD and Robert N. Weinreb, MD

WHY A NEW TEST IS NEEDED

Standard automated achromatic perimetry (white flash on white background) does not detect optic nerve damage at an early stage. There can be considerable structural change in the optic nerve head in eyes with glaucoma before additional visual field loss is detected by standard achromatic perimetry. Short-wavelength automated perimetry (SWAP) addresses these problems to some extent.

THE RATIONALE FOR SWAP

Loss of normal color vision is associated with glaucoma, and blue-green color vision deficits are apparent early in the disease process. This region of color vision is handled by the short-wavelength cones and their neural connections. For an unknown reason, glaucoma either affects this system early in the disease process or we are more able to detect early damage in this system. Evidence of blue-green deficits on cen-

Figure 9-1. The log relative spectral radiance of the violet stimulus (□) and yellow background (○) used in SWAP in watts/steradians/m² by nanometers (nm). The x axis spans the range of normal human vision from violet at 400 nm through blue, to blue-green, to green, to yellow, to orange, and red at 700 nm. These curves represent parameters agreed upon by several researchers and in use with the Humphrey Field Analyzers.

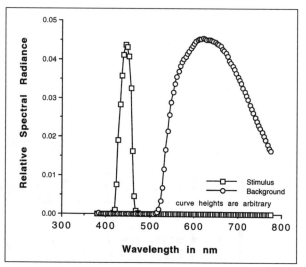

tral color vision tests such as the Farnsworth-Munsell 100 hue test, the Farnsworth D-15, and the Pickford-Nicholson anomaloscope is often present before peripheral visual field loss is found by standard perimetry. However, color vision screening tests are not useful for predicting the progress of the disease. Several factors other than glaucoma can affect these tests, such as lens density, pupil size, macular pigment, and other underlying medical diseases, such as diabetes. Even when these factors are controlled and significant differences between normal eyes and eyes with primary open-angle glaucoma can be documented, the separation between the groups is not sufficient for diagnosis and long-term management.

Two other factors that may have reduced the predictive ability of previous color vision testing in glaucoma are the emphasis on foveally presented (fixated) stimuli and the use of tests designed originally to assess congenital color vision deficits. Tests that isolate short-wavelength cone mechanisms and that exploit the known loss of peripheral visual field sensitivity are more appropriate for assessing eyes with primary open-angle glaucoma. SWAP was developed to incorporate this knowledge. By testing only the short-wavelength sensitive mechanisms throughout the central 30° visual field, we are reducing any redundancy in the system, which may allow detection of the stimulus through some other visual pathway. This is unlike the stimulus in standard achromatic perimetry, which may be detected by any one of several systems.

WHAT IS SWAP?

Short-wavelength automated perimetry is identical to standard achromatic automated perimetry except that it tests only an isolated part of the color vision system: the short-wavelength (blue) sensitive cones and their neural connections. The key parameters necessary to isolate the short-wavelength system are a broad bright yellow background wavelength range of approximately 500 to 750 nanometers (nm) inside the perimeter bowl and a Goldmann size V (1.8° visual angle) violet test target centered at a wavelength of 440 nm (Figure 9-1). The stimulus duration is 200 milliseconds (msec). The yellow background adapts the rods and the middle wavelength and long wavelength-sensitive cones so they are much less able to detect the violet test stimulus. The color of the stimulus is centered in the wavelength range where the short-wavelength cones can detect it best. With this set-up, an increase in stimulus intensity of approximately 15 decibels (dB) is required before any other component of the visual system can detect the stimulus.

HOW USEFUL IS SWAP FOR DIAGNOSIS AND MANAGEMENT OF GLAUCOMA?

Two independent prospective longitudinal studies of SWAP have indicated that the test is more sensitive for detecting early abnormalities than is standard achromatic automated perimetry, showing abnormal results two to five years prior to the development of abnormal standard visual fields in 83% of eyes. In other studies, SWAP successfully differentiated between normal and glaucoma eyes, and the prevalence of SWAP defects increased with increasing risk for glaucoma. The location of the short-wavelength visual field defects was often the same as that later detected with standard visual field testing. Additionally, in glaucoma eyes, short-wavelength fields have indicated more extensive damage across the retina than standard visual fields, and they have shown progressive loss one to three years sooner. SWAP results correlate well with structural measures of the optic nerve head, and the location of SWAP defects correspond well to the optic nerve head topography in patients with both defects. Preliminary studies have also shown SWAP to be effective for diagnosis and follow-up of visual field loss associated with diabetes and several neuro-ophthalmologic disorders and with secondary and normal-tension glaucomas.

PERFORMANCE OF SWAP ON THE HUMPHREY VISUAL FIELD ANALYZER

SWAP is now available on the Humphrey Visual Field Analyzer II. To access the SWAP version of a test (eg, 30-2, 24-2, neurological, etc), select the desired test and the test eye as usual. Enter the patient data. When the test display screen appears, select "change parameters." Select the "blue-yellow" option in the lower left corner of the screen, and then press "selection complete." When the test screen reappears, the words "non-standard parameters" should appear in the upper mid-right portion of the display under the test eye. Continue the test as usual. When the test is complete "save to disk" as usual.

Three print options are now available for SWAP: the single-field analysis, an overview of two or more fields, and a three-in-one, which gives the graytone, numeric decibels, and total deviation plots only. Each printout is designated as blue-yellow in the upper right-hand corner and also by the notations, "stimulus: V, blue, background yellow" (Figure 9-2). Reliability indices for fixation loss, false positive errors, false negative errors, and fluctuation are available on the printout, and gaze tracking is available. On rare occasions, testing the blind spot with a size V target is a problem, and the operator will need to either switch to a size III or turn the blind spot check off and monitor the fixation carefully by eye.

INTERPRETATION OF SWAP VISUAL FIELDS

With short-wavelength automated perimetry, both age and cataract can be taken into account and thresholds adjusted accordingly through the use of probability plots and statistical analyses, such as the Glaucoma Hemifield Test. These analyses are based on a large normative database and are currently available on newer Humphrey instruments. However, there are several additional factors unique to SWAP that we now know should also be taken into account when interpreting results. Some studies have shown that SWAP has similar test-retest reliability, short-term fluctuation, and long-term fluctuation to that found for standard perimetry, while others show increased variability and a longer learning curve for SWAP. New studies have also shown that the SWAP field in normal eyes has a steeper hill of vision (poorer sensitivity) in the superior visual field relative to the inferior field. The manufacturer has modified the statistical analysis package for SWAP to incorporate these new findings to improve the sensitivity of the comparisons between an individual patient's field and the normative database. Interpretation of SWAP fields, therefore, should only be made using the probability plots and not the threshold values or the grayscale. When an abnormality is found in a patient taking a SWAP test for the first time, a repeat field to verify the abnormality should be done. SWAP has also been shown to be valuable for diagnosis of several other neurological or retinal diseases, including diabetic retinopathy, optic neuritis, and HIV-related visual loss.

In summary, SWAP is a new commercially available visual field test that has been well-validated. It is more sensitive to early glaucomatous damage and more useful in monitoring progression when compared to standard perimetry. The planned further development by Humphrey of SITA-SWAP and associated statistical analysis packages should expand the clinical utility of SWAP for the glaucoma specialist.

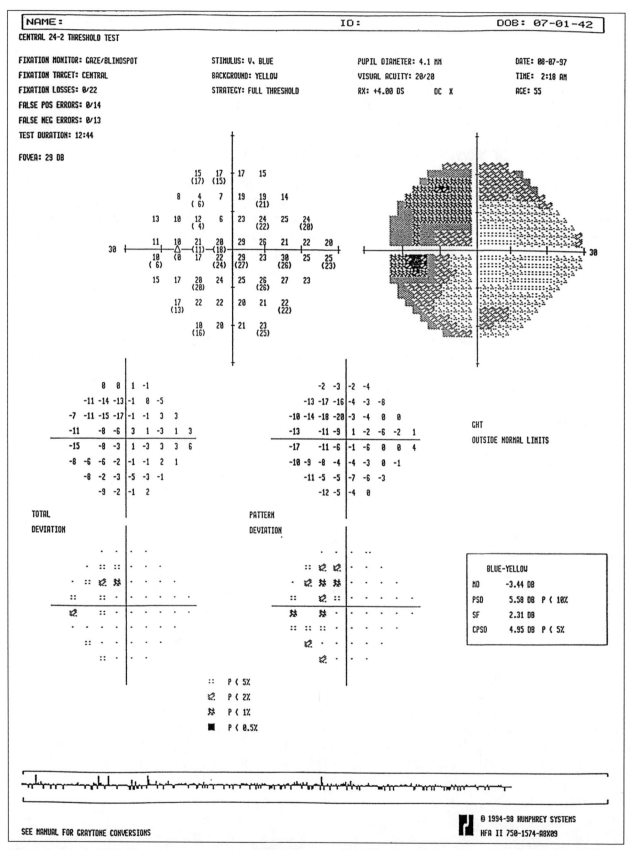

Figure 9-2. A single-field analysis printout of visual field results from the Humphrey Visual Field Analyzer II perimeter for a SWAP 24-2 program.

Swedish Interactive Thresholding Algorithm (SITA)

Boel Bengtsson, PhD and Anders Heijl, MD, PhD

RATIONALE FOR DEVELOPING SITA

Computerized perimetric threshold strategies are the most sensitive techniques for detecting glaucomatous loss of visual function and the most appropriate methods for perimetric follow-up of glaucoma patients. They make it possible to detect shallow depressions in tested fields. Results from such tests are suitable for statistical analyses, and valuable interpretation tools like probability maps have been developed for them. Unfortunately, threshold tests are rather time consuming. Long tests are impractical in clinical settings and often uncomfortable for patients. With the most ambitious test strategies (eg, the full threshold and 30-2 test point pattern), test durations up to 20 minutes per eye are seen in eyes with visual field loss. The FASTPAC strategy applies longer steps in stimulus staircases and fewer crossings of the threshold than the full threshold strategy. This results in shorter tests, but less reliable test data. In SITA, new computer-intensive techniques are used for threshold estimation. These made it possible to considerably shorten test times without decreasing the accuracy of test results as compared with current standard threshold tests. Two versions of SITA have been developed: SITA Standard and SITA Fast. SITA Standard was designed to replace the full threshold strategy, and SITA Fast replaced the FASTPAC strategy. The SITA strategies use the Humphrey standard test parameters (ie, Goldmann size III white stimuli on a white background).

METHODS USED IN SITA

The time-saving effects of SITA have been achieved using three different features:

1. Real-time calculation of threshold values and estimation of measurement errors in threshold values. This novelty is the main reason that it has been possible to shorten test times without decreasing the accuracy of test results. A visual field model that is used for calculation of threshold values during the actual test is already available before the start of the test. The model depends on patient age but is valid for all sorts of fields, normal as well as defective. Hence, it is important to enter the patient's birth date correctly before the test begins. This prior visual field model is based on frequency-of-seeing (FOS) curves, which describe probabilities for a stimulus of certain intensity to be perceived. Prospectively collected data of normal and glaucomatous fields, including FOS-curve measurements, were used to construct these prior visual field models.

   Threshold values at adjacent test points also influence the model, particularly if located along the same nerve fiber bundle.

   The actual visual field test starts by measuring threshold values at four primary points, one located in each of the four quadrants of the test point pattern, just as in traditional strategies. Threshold results at these primary points are used to determine starting intensities at a few adjacent points. As more test data become available, more points are opened for testing. All test points in the chosen test-point pattern are subjected to testing. Traditional bracketing methods are used. The visual field model changes continuously during the test and both threshold values and measurement errors in threshold values are repeatedly calculated from the model at all points during the test. After a minimum number of answers to stimulus exposures or threshold crossings, stimulus sequences can be interrupted, but only if measurement errors are small enough according to predefined levels of accuracy.

   Rules for interruption of stimulus sequences are different for SITA Standard and SITA Fast. SITA Standard requires smaller measurement errors than SITA Fast. During the development of SITA, these rules were defined with the help of computer simulations. The accuracy of SITA Standard test results was required to be the same or better than the full-threshold strategy. Similarly, SITA Fast was designed to surpass or equal the FASTPAC strategy.

2. New methods for estimating the reliability parameters of false negative and false positive answers. Traditionally, false positive and false negative answers are measured by adding extra questions to the test, called catch trials. The number of catch trials must be very limited so as not to unduly prolong the test. In SITA, catch trials are used only to estimate false negative answers, and then in combination with a new method that extracts data from patterns of patient responses immediately after the test is finished, during the post-processing of data. Test time is further shortened since catch trials are not used for estimation of frequencies of false positive answers. Instead, SITA uses a new method that records positive responses during periods in the test where no such answers are expected. One such period appears immediately at the onset of a stimulus exposure and lasts for 180 msec, where no true answers can possibly occur. The total sampling time during a test available for recording false positive answers is much longer than that available for sampling with traditional catch trials. False positive answers are also extracted from patterns of patients' responses during post-processing. Hence, the new methods to measure false positives are more precise than the old catch trial method. In this way, SITA can apply more effective methods to estimate false answers and simultaneously reduce test time.

3. An improved flexible timing algorithm for stimulus presentation is also used. The new timing algorithm follows the patient's pacing of button activity throughout the entire test by continuously recording the reaction time to perceived stimuli. Response windows are repeatedly calculated. During the post-processing of test results, all response intervals are checked and adjusted if necessary. Late answers regarded as not seen during the actual test can then be reclassified as seen and vice versa.

The calculation of threshold values and measurement errors in real time is the single most important factor for saving test time in SITA. Approximately 33% of test time is saved in SITA Standard and SITA Fast as compared with full threshold and FASTPAC respectively because of this feature alone. The new methods to estimate false answers and the new timing algorithm shorten test times by another 17% (approximately).

SITA IN CLINICAL PRACTICE

The SITA Standard strategy has been compared with the full threshold and the FASTPAC strategies in two clinical prospective studies—one study in normal subjects, the other in glaucoma patients. Test times were reduced by 50% on the average both in normal and in glaucoma patients, when using SITA Standard as compared with full threshold. SITA Standard was about 15% faster than FASTPAC.

SITA Fast was compared to the full threshold and FASTPAC strategies in another prospective study of glaucoma patients. Here, test times were further reduced by another 66% as compared with full threshold and 47% compared to FASTPAC (Figure 9-3).

Accuracy of test results are important but difficult to determine in clinical tests. In theory, true visual fields and true threshold values must be known to calculate accuracy. The "true" visual fields cannot be measured, however, since measured sensitivities are influenced by learning effects, visual fatigue, perimetrist influence, physiological variability, degree of glaucomatous visual field loss, etc. In clinical evaluations, one must therefore usually rely on test-retest variability, accepting the assumptions that test results obtained with a test strategy showing high reproducibility are likely to be more accurate than results obtained with another strategy showing low reproducibility.

In two studies, test-retest variability was slightly lower in tests obtained with SITA Standard than those obtained with full threshold. FASTPAC tests had the largest test-retest variability in both studies. In the SITA Fast study, test-retest variability was slightly lower with SITA Fast than with full threshold; again FASTPAC variability was slightly larger.

In grayscale printouts, field defects sometimes appear smaller and shallower in shorter tests than in longer ones. This is particularly obvious in the shortest tests (ie, those obtained with SITA Fast). This is explained by the small degree of visual fatigue in tests as short as SITA Fast. Visual fatigue is known to cause diminished sensitivity with increasing test time, particularly at test points located close to points with deep defects. By using interpretation tools, SITA STATPAC probability maps, instead of grayscales when judging test results, such differences between short and long tests are largely eliminated.

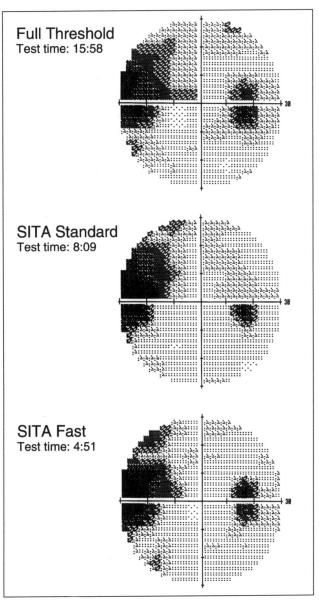

Figure 9-3. Test results of the same eye obtained with the three different strategies: full threshold, SITA Standard, and SITA Fast. Grayscale printouts appear similar, but test times were significantly different.

The statistical analysis package STATPAC is now available for SITA. Visual field data from normal subjects collected at several eye centers all over the world were used. Test strategies with small intersubject variability give narrower limits for normality than those with large intersubject variability. Hence, low intersubject variability improves detection of shallow visual field defects. Both SITA Standard and SITA Fast have narrower limits for normality than full threshold and FASTPAC. This means that STATPAC probability maps for SITA can provide much more important information about the field status than grayscale printouts alone (Figure 9-4).

In grayscale printouts, shallow but significant depressions located in areas with high sensitivity and low normal intersubject variability may be invisible (Figure 9-5). The opposite may also be seen. Regions in grayscales appearing suspect or pathological can very well be within the normal range if located in areas with high normal variability (Figure 9-6).

The high reproducibility of SITA test results will increase the ability to detect small changes in series of fields. This will be visible, for example, in the glaucoma change probability maps, which are currently under development for SITA.

Figure 9-4. Grayscale printouts and pattern deviation probability maps from an eye tested with full threshold, SITA Standard, and SITA Fast. In the grayscales, the visual field defect is obvious with full threshold and barely visible with SITA Fast. In probability maps, the defect appears distinctly with all three strategies.

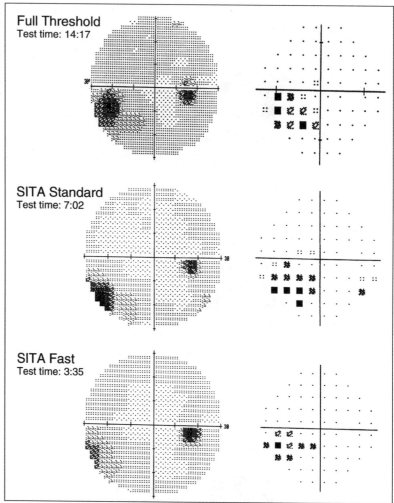

The Humphrey Field Analyzer and SITA

The two SITA strategies, SITA Standard and SITA Fast, are available in the Humphrey Field Analyzer II perimeters. These SITA programs are based on visual field models using standard test parameters (ie, white stimuli on white background and Goldmann stimulus size III). SITA Standard and SITA Fast are available for the standard test point patterns 30-2, 24-2, and on the central 10-2 and peripheral 60-4. STATPAC limits are available for 30-2, 24-2, and 10-2. SITA Standard is normally the default in the HFA II and is thereby preselected. Check with your Humphrey Systems representative. To access the SITA strategies, select the desired test point pattern and test eye as usual. When the test screen appears, select "change parameters." Choose the "strategy" menu in the upper left corner and highlight the "SITA Standard" or "SITA Fast" option, and then select "return." When the test screen reappears, the chosen strategy is visible in the upper right part of the display. It is also possible to choose one of the SITA strategies as standard by selecting "system set-up" from the main menu and select "alter main menu."

Further Applications with SITA

SITA is not yet available for SWAP, but it is under development. This requires a new visual field model based on SWAP normal data, pathological test results, and FOS measurements.

SITA in the Future

It is also possible to use the SITA concept with other tests using different stimulus color, stimulus size, or with almost any other thresholding techniques. New visual field models based on empirical data must then

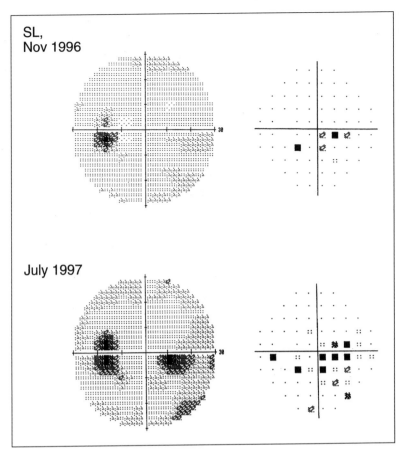

Figure 9-5. Grayscale and pattern deviation probability map printouts of a glaucomatous visual field. Top: The test result appears rather normal in the grayscale printout, but an inferior arcuate defect is present in the probability map. Bottom: The same eye tested seven months later; the defect is now seen in grayscale maps.

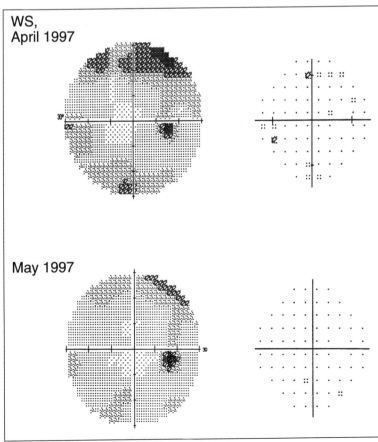

Figure 9-6. Two test results from a normal eye obtained within a few weeks. Top: Some questionable dark areas in the grayscale printout, possibly caused by lack of perimetric experience or patient fatigue. The probability maps are essentially normal. Bottom: At the following examination, grayscale and probability maps both appear normal.

be constructed in order to exploit the increased efficacy that the SITA concept can provide. This involves a great deal of perimetric research since a new STATPAC version must be developed for each new test type. It is, therefore, realistic to assume that such modifications will be implemented only if they are believed to be of clear benefit clinically.

Kinetic Perimetry

Some of the principles of kinetic perimetry were discussed in Chapter 1. Performing an examination on the Goldmann perimeter requires a well-trained technician and is a labor-intensive process. A properly performed examination for glaucoma, for example, requires identification of a suprathreshold stimulus at 25° temporally (5° above or below the horizontal meridian), mapping the blind spot, and a peripheral isopter with that stimulus using the kinetic technique of moving the stimulus (manually) with the shutter open from areas of non-seeing toward seeing areas (ie, from the center of the blind spot outward and from the periphery toward the center), mapping two or more additional isopters, usually one centrally and one peripherally (requiring the technician to choose the appropriate stimulus size and intensity), verification of all identified steps by movement of the stimulus perpendicularly to the axes, static searches for central and paracentral scotomata, and finally, detailed mapping of all identified scotomata. Remember that kinetic testing does not give a topographical map of the island of vision; rather, it generates a top-down view of the island showing the boundaries of areas of equal or greater sensitivity. Should kinetic testing be desired, the Humphrey perimeter (with appropriate software) is capable of performing a semi-automatic kinetic test. The process for this is detailed in its user's manual. A few key points are in order:

1. The default stimulus is the I2E, and the machine does not do an automated determination of the suprathreshold stimulus intensity needed for the first isopter (the default can be changed, if desired).
2. The operator must select additional isopters to be tested since they are not determined automatically (up to 10 isopters can be plotted per eye). Scotomata can only be mapped if the operator pinpoints the starting location for the map. Central and paracentral scotomata can be searched for statically in custom scan mode by selecting the pad labeled "static test currently off" (it will then be turned on). The operator must then manually select each point to be tested statically, and that point will have a one-second stimulus presentation. Any points not seen can then be explored as indicated above. Fixation behavior is not automatically monitored—the operator must watch the image of the eye on the video eye monitor for shifts in fixation (the image will move around the screen so as not to block out the image of the moving target).
3. Finally, printing can only be done on the internal dot matrix printer. If a laser printer is attached to the serial port, the machine will print the kinetic test on the dot matrix printer and then reset the system to the laser.

Kinetic perimetry on the Humphrey perimeter requires a technician with the skills and knowledge required to perform Goldmann perimetry. This test modality is not automated in the same manner as threshold testing, and all the machine does in essence is control the movement of the projector, the opening of the shutter, record the patient responses, and plot the results. The test is highly interactive with the technician. Figure 9-7 is an example of a kinetic test performed on the Humphrey perimeter. The test was performed by a perimetrist not familiar with Goldmann testing. Only a single isopter was plotted using the default I2E stimulus. The top of the figure shows what appears to be a vertical step. The blind spot was not mapped, nor were static searches conducted for scotomata. The bottom of the figure shows the other printout option for kinetic tests, that is, a numerical printout listing each meridian tested, the starting and stopping point for the projector (degrees from fixation along that meridian for start and stop as well as the X, Y coordinates of the start and stop points), the isopter tested, the patient response, and the test type (standard or static).

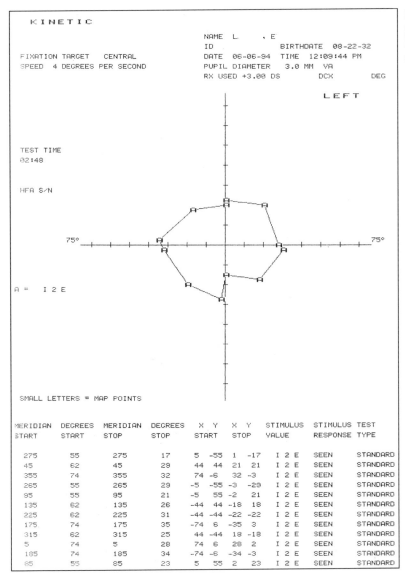

Figure 9-7. Top: Single isopter kinetic field plot from the Humphrey Field Analyzer. Bottom: Numerical printout from kinetic examination.

MERIDIAN START	DEGREES START	MERIDIAN STOP	DEGREES STOP	X START	Y START	X STOP	Y STOP	STIMULUS VALUE	STIMULUS RESPONSE	TEST TYPE
275	55	275	17	5	-55	1	-17	I 2 E	SEEN	STANDARD
45	62	45	29	44	44	21	21	I 2 E	SEEN	STANDARD
355	74	355	32	74	-6	32	-3	I 2 E	SEEN	STANDARD
265	55	265	29	-5	-55	-3	-29	I 2 E	SEEN	STANDARD
95	55	95	21	-5	55	-2	21	I 2 E	SEEN	STANDARD
135	62	135	26	-44	44	-18	18	I 2 E	SEEN	STANDARD
225	62	225	31	-44	-44	-22	-22	I 2 E	SEEN	STANDARD
175	74	175	35	-74	6	-35	3	I 2 E	SEEN	STANDARD
315	62	315	25	44	-44	18	-18	I 2 E	SEEN	STANDARD
5	74	5	28	74	6	28	2	I 2 E	SEEN	STANDARD
185	74	185	34	-74	-6	-34	-3	I 2 E	SEEN	STANDARD
85	55	85	23	5	55	2	23	I 2 E	SEEN	STANDARD

Analytical Software Packages

STATPAC and STATPAC 2 have been discussed previously in Chapters 1 and 5. Other software packages are available, offering alternative methods for displaying and analyzing data from Humphrey threshold tests. Please note that information contained in this section changes rapidly and may not be correct or applicable to your particular machine model. See your Zeiss-Humphrey representative for the latest information.

PATIENTVIEW FIELD PRESENTATION SOFTWARE

PatientView is a software package available from Humphrey Instruments that enables an IBM-compatible personal computer to read data from Humphrey floppy disks or download fields from the perimeter via the serial port and display the information on the computer screen. The fields may then be printed on an Epson FX-80 compatible dot matrix printer, an HP LaserJet II/III laser printer, or Postscript-equipped laser printer. The program runs under DOS version 3.3 or 5.0, and is not recommended for running under Microsoft Windows™. The software will display value tables, total deviation plots from expected age-matched normals, graytone, graytone with numeric data overlay (this display cannot be printed), and a three-dimensional surface or island of vision.

Figure 9-8. Example of three-dimensional island of vision map from PatientView field presentation software.

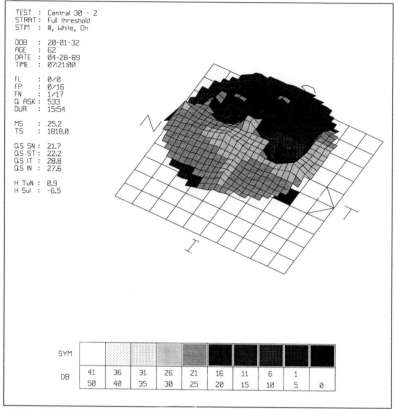

SYM									
DB	41	36	31	26	21	16	11	6	1
50	40	35	30	25	20	15	10	5	0

Figure 9-8 is an example of a three-dimensional surface printout from the PatientView field presentation software. This is the same field as Figure 1-12. The island of vision has been rotated and tilted to match the three-dimensional topographic map generated for that field. The test information is displayed in the upper left-hand corner of the printout. Additional information is provided at the bottom of the information window that is not available on standard printouts, including mean sensitivity, total sensitivity, quadrant sensitivity for each quadrant, and hemifield analysis (temporal versus nasal, superior versus inferior).

PatientView can be used with the 30-2, 24-2, and 10-2 threshold tests, the central 40-, 76-, and 80-point screening tests, the full-field 120-point screening test, and the peripheral 68-point screening test. The central 76-point test may be displayed as a three-dimensional surface. Multiple fields may be viewed simultaneously in separate windows, or two fields may be compared directly using a "dual" window. Additional information may be obtained from your Humphrey Instruments representative.

STATPAC for Windows

The cathode ray tube (CRT) of the Humphrey perimeter has limited capability for displaying visual field results and the results of data analysis. The viewing of multiple fields at a time is limited to printouts only since multiple fields cannot be displayed on the CRT. Data management, such as locating particular visual field results, is cumbersome due to the user interface and the need to scroll through disk contents one page at a time. STATPAC for Windows (SFW) is a software option offered by Humphrey Instruments that allows visual field data viewing and analysis using a DOS-based IBM-compatible personal computer, running Microsoft Windows™.

The SFW program is installed on the personal computer from floppy disks supplied with the package. A floppy disk drive is required in order to read data from the perimeter or else data must be transmitted to the computer through the perimeter's serial port. The program includes options for configuring the serial port of the computer to receive data from the perimeter. The Humphrey system uses a proprietary floppy disk formatting. Data stored on floppy disks cannot normally be read by a personal computer. In order to use field data from the perimeter with SFW, the data must be saved in a manner that will allow the SFW program to read it from the floppy disks. The software to make this configuration is contained in the machine's EPROMs. Therefore, the operating chips must be changed to make field data readable by the program. The chips are supplied with the purchase of the SFW package. Once installed, a new pad appears on the "disk functions" menu of the main menu that reads "configure floppy disk for STATPAC for Windows." This pad does not affect any data on the floppy disk except to make it readable by the SFW program. The data on the floppy disk must then be imported into SFW—the "import" button that appears on the button bar when SFW is opened will prompt for the insertion of a disk. The program then reads the disk and offers the option of selecting all files or individual files using the computer's pointing device. All selected fields are then imported into one large file called "statpac.dat."

SFW is started as any Windows program would be. A blank screen appears with a menu bar (file, records, charts, options, and help) and a button bar (import, open, print, right, left, prev, next, multi, and graph/num). Selecting the "open" button displays a list of all patients on the hard drive—only data on the hard drive can be opened. Once a patient is selected, a list of the available visual fields is displayed. Clicking "OK" will open all of the fields for that patient, and up to six graytone images will be displayed on the screen, arranged chronologically from earliest to latest left to right and top to bottom in a "graphic multititle raw threshold" chart. The right/left buttons toggle between right and left eye data. Both graphic and numeric multititle views are available, and each can be displayed as raw threshold, total deviation, pattern deviation, or global index views by selecting from the "chart" drop down menu or by clicking the appropriate button. Multititle views cannot be printed. Individual fields can be selected for view by clicking on them, and any of the STATPAC printouts can be displayed on the screen, including the single-field analysis, the three-in-one chart, the overview printout, the change analysis, and the glaucoma change probability. All of these charts can be printed. SFW does not print double-determined thresholds, but rather prints the average of repeat measurements. The examples that follow were printed on an HP LaserJet 4Si, with a resolution of 300 dots per inch (DPI). The graytones would appear more like the standard graytone if the printer could be set to a lower resolution, for example, 150 DPI. Therefore, the appearance of the graytones in these examples is not representative of what they should look like.

Figure 9-9 is a visual field result printed from SFW. This is the SFW three-in-one printout of the same visual field and patient shown in Figures 1-12 through 1-18 (Figure 1-12 is the value table, 1-14 is the defect depth, 1-15 is the graytone, and 1-16 is the standard three-in-one printout). Figure 9-10 is the SFW printout and analysis of this field (Figure 1-18 is the comparable standard STATPAC printout).

One addition to the SFW printouts is the little box under the glaucoma hemifield test (on the right side of the printout beneath the graytone) with an indicator for the degree of abnormality. All of the change over time printouts have this indicator for each field. Figure 9-11 is the first page of the overview analysis for this eye, and Figure 9-12 is the change analysis for all fields. SFW draws the lines connecting all plotted points.

Finally, Figure 9-13 is representative of the glaucoma change probability plot for the first three examinations in the series. In actuality, SFW begins the follow-up examinations on the next page; this figure has been cut and pasted to illustrate the appearance of the printout. The explanation for the glaucoma change probability symbols appears at the bottom of the last page of the actual printout (not shown in Figure 9-13).

FIELDVIEW OMEGA FROM VISMED/DICON

The Dicon TKS 4000 Autoperimeter is an automated static threshold perimeter that contains limited data manipulation capability. FieldView software was developed to allow the retrieval of patient data from floppy disks into a personal computer and to offer alternative visual field data displays to the printed output from the perimeter's internal printer. The current version of the software, called Omega, incorporates multiple display tools and age-related normal values for Dicon data. The software is also capable of reading Humphrey disks and displaying Humphrey visual fields in a variety of interesting ways. The software does not incorporate age-related normal values for Humphrey data; therefore, analysis is limited to the hill of vision (shape) model.

The FieldView Omega program runs under DOS but does not use the Windows graphical interface. It does, however, allow display of multiple fields in their own windows, which can be individually manipulat-

Figure 9-9. Three-in-one printout from STATPAC for Windows. (See text for explanation of printing methods and appearance of grayscale in this and subsequent examples).

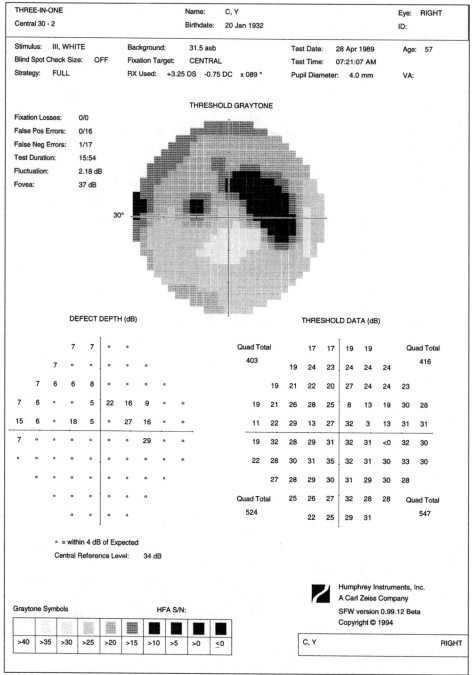

ed. When the program is loaded, a menu appears across the top of the screen with choices for fields (retrieve from hard disk or floppy), disk ID (label patient disk), displays (screen appearance), computer (setting perimeter options, printer set-up, FieldView options, patient diskette formatting), and quit. Arranged vertically along the left side of the screen are various icons showing the options for displaying the data. These are shown in Figure 9-14. They are, from top to bottom, numerical threshold values, grayscale, 3-D hill of vision, profile, ranked order, histogram, and isopters. A printer icon appears in the lower left-hand corner of the screen. The full screen or just one window can be printed.

Figure 9-15 shows the data display of a field retrieved from a Humphrey floppy disk in this full screen printout. This is the same visual field illustrated using SFW and in Chapter 1. Abnormal values appear (on the screen) in different colors according to their significance of abnormality. The P values corresponding to the colors are listed on the left side of the screen below the icons. At the top of the field window are two small

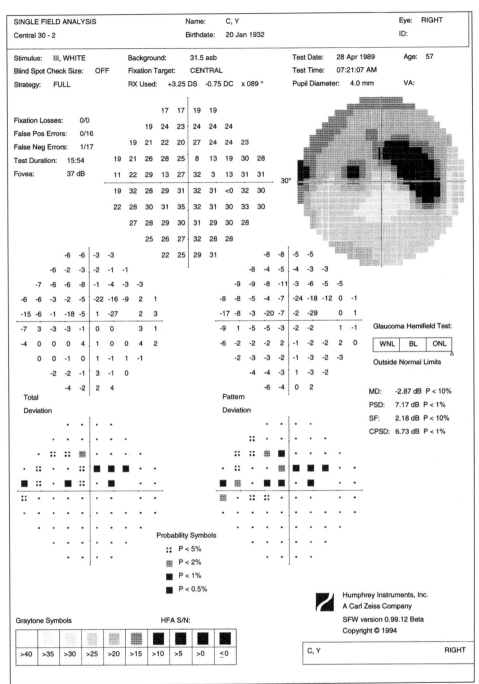

Figure 9-10. Single field analysis printout from STATPAC for Windows.

icons. The one with the question mark accesses context sensitive help. The icon with the three horizontal lines brings up a submenu, as illustrated. Patient information and test conditions (reliability, fluctuation, etc) can be viewed. The lower right-hand corner of the window contains a display icon. Clicking this icon will change the type of display. The display can be changed three ways: from the icon bar on the left side of the screen, from the icon in the lower right-hand corner of the field window, and from the "graphs" submenu. Figure 9-16 shows the grayscale view of this field. The FieldView Omega software grayscale uses a three-decibel increment scale. Clicking the box just below the test date allows the raw threshold data to be superimposed on the grayscale, as shown in Figure 9-17. The 3-D hill of vision creates a three-dimensional view of the island of vision and is displayed in Figure 9-18. The three-dimensional view can be rotated and tilted to allow multiple views. Figure 9-19 shows the island rotated and tilted slightly down to allow a view directly into the scotoma canyon. Compare this to Figure 1-13. The isopter view (Figure 9-20) draws boundaries around the

Figure 9-11. Overview analysis from STATPAC for Windows.

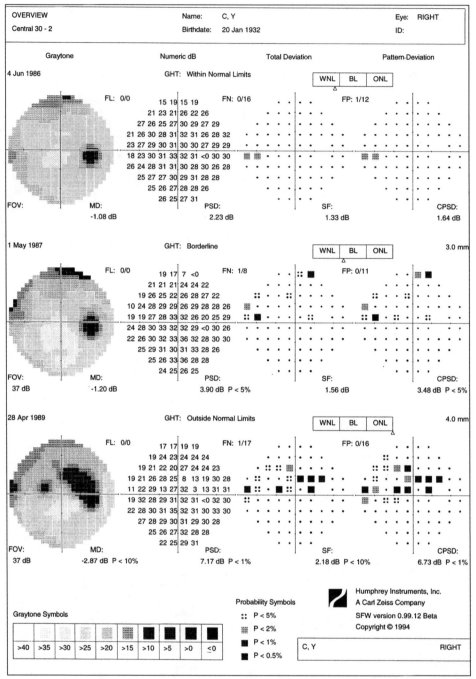

threshold data, resembling a Goldmann field. The user can pick which isopter to display by dragging the small box in the scroll bar on the left of the window.

FieldView Omega allows you to open up to four field windows. Each field can be displayed with a different view or all with the same view. Figures 9-21 (grayscale) and 9-22 (3-D island of vision) show one prior and two subsequent fields from the series of fields containing the one in Figures 9-14 through 9-20.

FieldView Omega can perform a "delta" analysis between any two fields. One such analysis is shown in Figure 9-23. Points showing no change are indicated by a check mark, and a triangle symbol demonstrates points that are more than five decibels below expected normal. Red triangles signify points more than five decibels below normal in both tests, while green or blue triangles indicate points more than five decibels below normal in only one of the tests, the color matching the background color of the test containing the abnormal value.

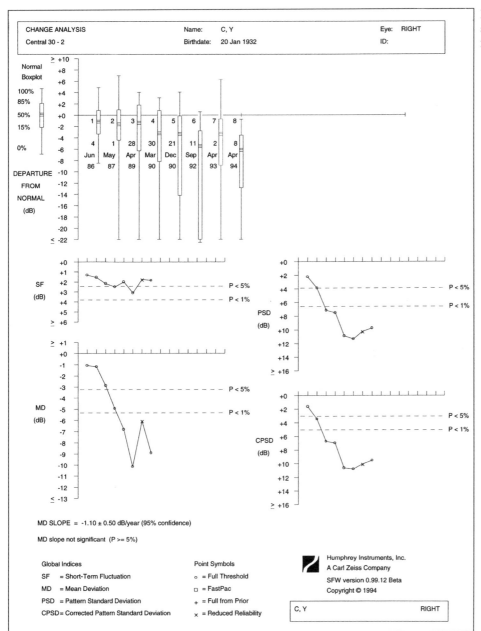

Figure 9-12. Change analysis printout from STATPAC for Windows.

An explanation of any aspect of FieldView Omega is available by clicking the question mark at the upper left of the window. The explanation of the meaning of the triangles appears in a separate window and is shown in Figure 9-24.

A delta analysis between two fields can also be displayed with a numerical difference plot. This plot can have the threshold difference between all points (Figure 9-25) or display only points that have changed, labeled "Diff Only" (Figure 9-26).

PeriData Visual Field Management Software

Peridata is a software package from Interzeag, Inc for IBM-compatible personal computers. This company manufactures and distributes the Octopus™ line of automated perimeters. Peridata is designed to allow the viewing and analysis of visual field data from both the Octopus and Humphrey perimeters in a standardized format. The package contains a full library of statistical programs and the ability to accept raw data from either perimeter. It can be used as an alternative to STATPAC. All familiar displays and printouts are avail-

Figure 9-13. Glaucoma change probability plot printout from STATPAC for Windows.

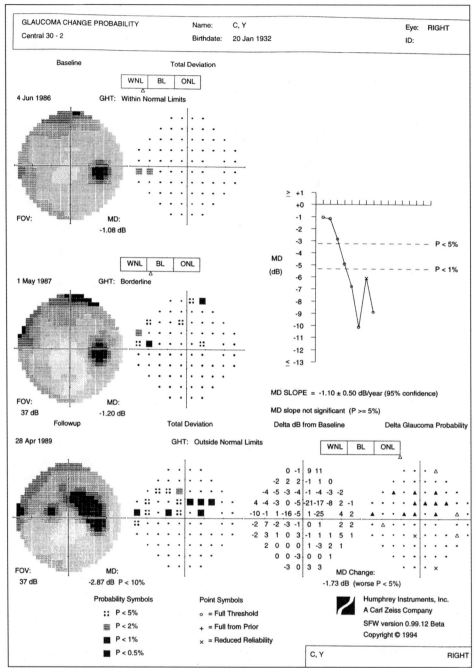

able, and some other data presentation formats have been added, including color three-dimensional displays of the island of vision, cumulative defect curves (Bebie curve), stack bar analyses, graphical analyses of topographical trends, graphical analyses of numerical trends, and long-term overview trend analyses.

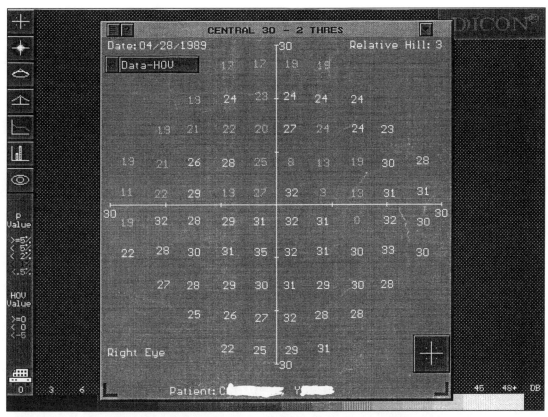

Figure 9-14. Full screen printout showing the threshold data window from FieldView Omega.

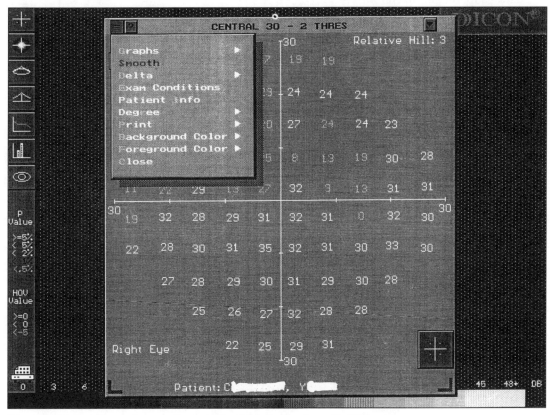

Figure 9-15. Options submenu for a single-field display from FieldView Omega.

Figure 9-16. Window printout of a grayscale display from FieldView Omega.

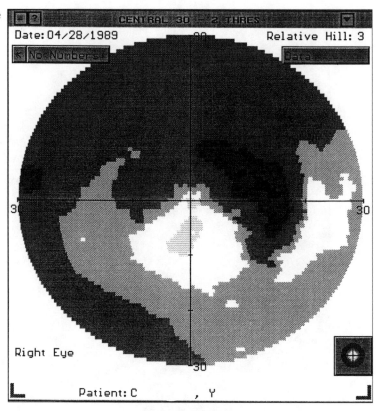

Figure 9-17. Single field window with numeric data superimposed on a grayscale from FieldView Omega.

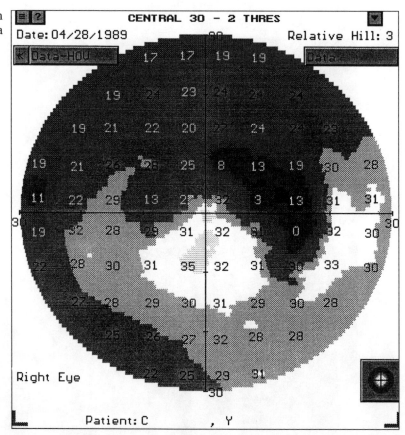

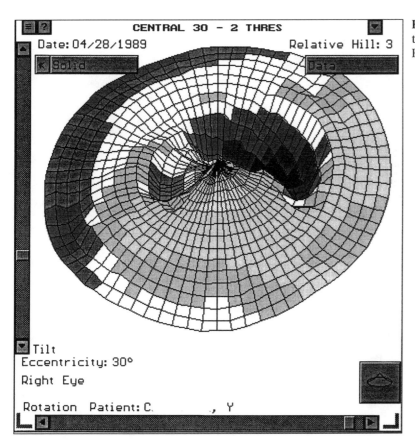

Figure 9-18. Single field window with three-dimensional island of vision from FieldView Omega.

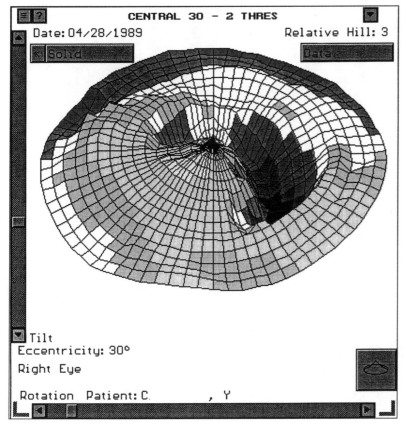

Figure 9-19. Three-dimensional island of vision rotated to match Figure 1-13.

Figure 9-20. Single field window with isopters from FieldView Omega.

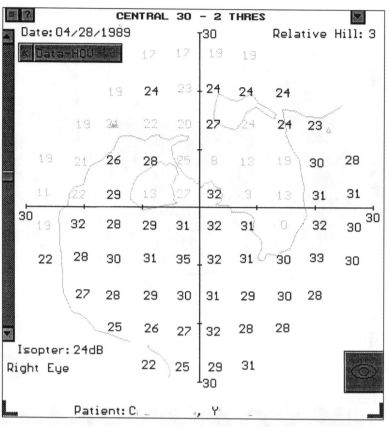

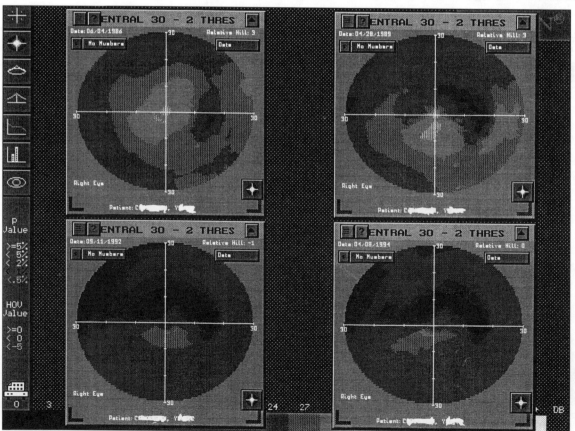

Figure 9-21. Multiple windows showing grayscales of four consecutive visual fields of the same patient from FieldView Omega.

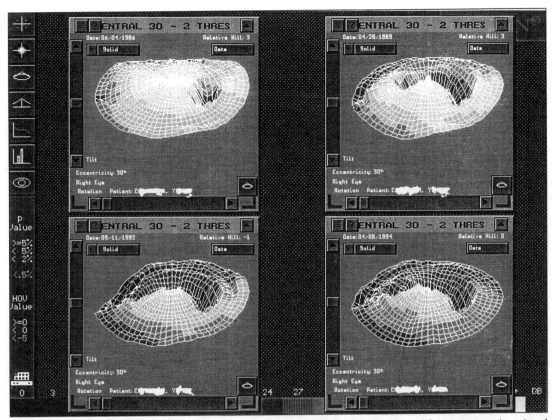

Figure 9-22. Multiple windows showing three-dimensional islands of vision of four consecutive visual fields of the same patient from FieldView Omega.

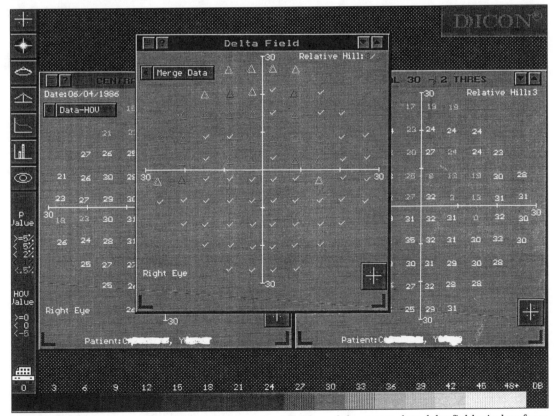

Figure 9-23. Full screen printout showing two visual fields and the merge data delta field window from FieldView Omega.

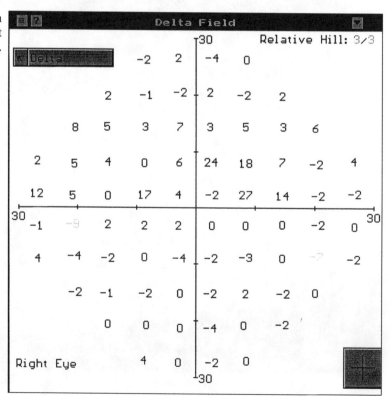

> **TRIANGLES**
>
> On the TKS plots, LD printouts and FieldView displays and printouts, Check Marks signify points tested and seen by the patient in SUPRATHRESHOLD and QMP (Quantify Missed Points) exams, or points seen in both fields of a DELTA MERGE view.
>
> Triangles signify points missed twice in Suprathreshold exams, or points more than 5 DECIBELS below EXPECTED NORMAL in either or both fields in a Delta Merge view, or points missed once in a BLIND SPOT MAPPING.
>
> Triangles will appear in different colors depending on the type of field display:
>
> - Red in Suprathreshold exams, or the same points that are more than 5dB below expected normal in both fields in a DELTA MERGE view.
>
> - Green or Blue when more than 5dB below expected normal in only one of two fields in a Delta Merge view. Here the color matches the background color of the field in which the point was missed.
>
> See also: PLOT CHECK MARKS, RED NUMBERS
>
> [Index] [Close]

Figure 9-24. Example help screen explaining the meaning of the triangle in Figure 9-16 from FieldView Omega.

Figure 9-25. Delta field window from FieldView Omega showing point-by-point numerical differences between the two fields.

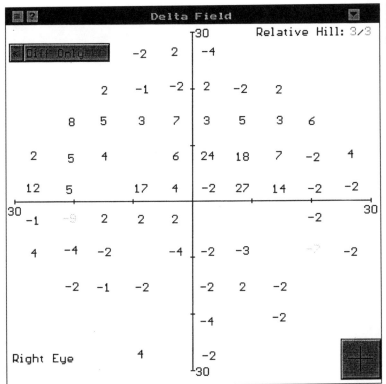

Figure 9-26. Delta field window from FieldView Omega showing the difference only window.

Appendix

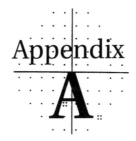

A

Visual Field Examples, by Diagnosis

DIAGNOSIS	MAIN FINDING	EXAMINATION TYPE	FIGURE NUMBER
	weak projector bulb	threshold	2-3
	nondiagnostic	screening	2-6
	nondiagnostic	screening	4-1
	incorrect birth date	threshold	4-13
	sample three in one printout	threshold	5-1
	white scotomata, high false positives	threshold	5-2
	white scotomata, 90% false positives	threshold	5-3
	white scotomata, 100% false positives	threshold	5-4
	100% false negatives	threshold	5-6
	high fixation loss due to incorrect fixation	threshold	5-7
	normal exam	threshold	5-16
	sample STATPAC printout	threshold	5-25
Artifact	diffuse loss of sensitivity, tested without add	threshold	4-15
	lens holder artifact	threshold	4-21
	lens holder artifact	threshold	5-12
	lens holder artifact	threshold	5-13
	correcting lens artifact	threshold	5-14
	correcting lens artifact	threshold	5-15
	pupillary effects	threshold	5-17
	diffuse depression, incorrect lens power	threshold	5-18
	diffuse depression, correcting lens power	threshold	5-20L
	diffuse depression,	threshold	5-20R

DIAGNOSIS	MAIN FINDING	EXAMINATION TYPE	FIGURE NUMBER
	correcting lens power		
	diffuse loss from incorrect correcting lens	threshold	5-21
	graytone construction artifact	threshold	5-22
	diffuse depression, graytone artifact	threshold	5-23
Cataract	diffuse depression	threshold	5-24
	diffuse depression	threshold	5-32
	worsening then improvement	threshold	5-37
	diffuse depression	threshold	8-9
Cerebrovascular accident	homonymous hemianopia	screening	4-5
	homonymous hemianopia	threshold	4-6
	quadrantanopia	threshold	7-29
Chiasmal inflammation, multiple sclerosis	bitemporal hemianopia	threshold	7-24
Cilioretinal artery occlusion	arcuate scotoma	threshold	8-18
Congenital optic nerve pit	nerve fiber bundle defect	threshold	8-5
Congenitally aberrant optic nerve	enlargement of the blind spot	threshold	8-1
	enlargement of the blind spot	threshold	8-2
	temporal nerve fiber bundle defect	threshold	8-3
	temporal nerve fiber bundle defect	threshold	8-4
Diabetic retinopathy, macular edema	diffuse loss of sensitivity, central scotoma	threshold	8-19
Encephalomalacia	quadrantanopia	threshold	7-28
Grave's disease	diffuse loss	threshold	7-16
Hypertensive crisis	central scotomata	threshold	8-20
	central scotomata	threshold	8-21
	peripheral loss	threshold	8-22
Ischemic optic neuropathy	altitudinal hemianopia	threshold	7-8
	altitudinal hemianopia	threshold	7-9
Juvenile glaucoma	nasal step	threshold	4-14
	nasal step	threshold	5-25
	nasal step	threshold	6-8
	end stage loss	threshold	6-16
	progressive nasal loss	threshold	6-22
Laser injury	paracentral defect	threshold	8-11
	paracentral defect	threshold	8-12
Left parietal lobe epidermoid cyst	homonymous hemianopia	screening	1-11
Low tension glaucoma	arcuate scotoma, value table	threshold	1-12
	arcuate scotoma, defect depth	threshold	1-14
	arcuate scotoma, graytone	threshold	1-15
	arcuate scotoma, profile	threshold	1-16
	altitudinal defect	threshold	6-14
	far advanced loss	threshold	6-15
	progressive nerve fiber loss	threshold	6-19
	progressive glaucomatous loss, new defects	threshold	6-23
	progressive low tension glaucoma	threshold	6-24
Macular degeneration	central scotoma	threshold	8-25
Macular hole	central scotoma	threshold	8-26

DIAGNOSIS	MAIN FINDING	EXAMINATION TYPE	FIGURE NUMBER
Melanocytoma	nerve fiber bundle defect	threshold	8-8
Metastatic lung cancer	homonymous hemianopia	threshold	7-27a
	homonymous hemianopia	threshold	7-27b
Neuroretinitis (cat scratch disease)	cecocentral scotoma	threshold	8-28a
Nonphysiologic loss	peripheral constriction	threshold	7-30
Occipital lobe infarction	homonymous hemianopia	threshold	7-26
	homonymous hemianopia	threshold	7-26
Open-angle glaucoma	nerve fiber bundle defect	threshold	2-10
	nerve fiber bundle defect	threshold	2-10
	nerve fiber bundle defect	threshold	2-11
	altitudinal hemianopia	screening	4-2
	minimal superior loss	threshold	4-7
	nerve fiber bundle defect	threshold	4-8
	high false negatives	threshold	5-5
	high fluctuation	threshold	5-8
	high fluctuation	threshold	5-9
	arcuate scotoma	threshold	5-11
	pupil effect	threshold	5-17
	diffuse depression	threshold	5-26
	paracentral defect, nasal step	threshold	5-30
	abnormally high sensitivity	threshold	5-31
	arcuate scotoma	threshold	5-33
	progressive nasal loss, overview	threshold	5-34
	progressive nasal loss, glaucoma change	threshold	5-36
	nerve fiber bundle defect	threshold	5-38L
	nasal step	threshold	5-38R
	asymmetric depression	threshold	6-1
	diffuse loss of sensitivity	threshold	6-2
	paracentral scotoma	threshold	6-4
	arcuate scotoma	threshold	6-5
	arcuate scotoma	threshold	6-6
	inferior paracentral defect, nasal step	threshold	6-7
	arcuate scotoma	threshold	6-9
	temporal wedge defects	threshold	6-10
	nerve fiber bundle defect	threshold	6-11
	nerve fiber bundle defect	threshold	6-12R
	nerve fiber bundle defect	threshold	6-12L
	double arcuate scotoma	threshold	6-13
	progressive diffuse loss	threshold	6-17
	progressive glaucomatous loss, new defects	threshold	6-18
	new and progressive nerve fiber bundle defect	threshold	6-20
	progressive glaucomatous defects	threshold	6-21
Optic atrophy	end stage disease	threshold	4-9
	end stage disease, stimulus V required	threshold	4-10
	end stage disease	threshold	4-11
	central scotoma	threshold	7-12
	nerve fiber bundle defects	screening	8-7

DIAGNOSIS	MAIN FINDING	EXAMINATION TYPE	FIGURE NUMBER
Optic disc drusen	inferior loss	threshold	7-1a
	disc based loss	threshold	7-2
	peripheral constriction	threshold	7-3
	nasal step	threshold	8-6
Optic nerve meningioma	peripheral constriction	threshold	7-13
Optic neuritis	nasal loss	threshold	7-10R
	diffuse depression	threshold	7-10L
	diffuse depression	threshold	7-11
Papilledema	disc based loss	threshold	7-5
	enlargement of the blind spot	threshold	7-6
Parieto-occipital mass	homonymous hemianopia	threshold	7-25
Pituitary tumor	homonymous hemianopia	screening	2-7
	homonymous hemianopia	screening	2-8
	hemianopia	screening	2-9
	homonymous hemianopia	screening	4-3
	homonymous hemianopia	screening	4-4
	bitemporal hemianopia	threshold	7-18L
	bitemporal hemianopia	threshold	7-18R
	bitemporal hemianopia	threshold	7-19
	junctional scotoma	threshold	7-21
	homonymous hemianopia	threshold	7-22
Post-traumatic glaucoma	high fluctuation	threshold	6-3
Ptosis	lid artifact	threshold	5-10
	lid artifact	threshold	8-10
Retinal detachment	peripheral loss	threshold	8-27
Retinitis pigmentosa	ring scotoma	threshold	8-30R
	ring scotoma	threshold	8-30L
	ring scotoma	threshold	8-31a
	ring scotoma	threshold	8-31b
Rod-cone dystrophy	ring scotoma	threshold	8-29
Secondary glaucoma	diffuse depression, incorrect lens	threshold	5-18
	nasal step	threshold	5-19
Shock optic neuropathy	bilateral arcuate scotomata	threshold	8-17
Syphilitic optic neuritis	peripheral constriction	threshold	8-16
Toxoplasmosis	arcuate scotoma	threshold	8-15
Trauma	bitemporal hemianopia	threshold	7-23
	central loss, temporal wedge	threshold	8-13
	altitudinal hemianopia	threshold	8-14
	altitudinal hemianopia	screening	8-14

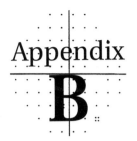

Appendix
B

Visual Field Examples, by Main Finding

MAIN FINDING	EXAMINATION TYPE	ARRAY USED	FIGURE NUMBER
100% false negatives	threshold	30-2	5-6
Abnormally high sensitivity	threshold	30-2	5-31
Altitudinal defect	threshold	30-2	6-14
Altitudinal hemianopia	screening	76 point	4-2
	threshold	30-2	7-8
	threshold	30-2	7-9
	threshold	30-2	8-14
	screening	120 point	8-14
Arcuate scotoma	threshold	30-2	5-11
	threshold	30-2	5-33
	threshold	30-2	6-5
	threshold	30-2	6-6
	threshold	30-2	6-9
	threshold	30-2	8-15
	threshold	30-2	8-18
Arcuate scotoma, defect depth	threshold	30-2	1-14
Arcuate scotoma, graytone	threshold	30-2	1-15
Arcuate scotoma, profile	threshold	30-2	1-16
Arcuate scotoma, value table	threshold	30-2	1-12
Asymmetric depression	threshold	30-2	6-1
Bilateral arcuate scotomata	threshold	30-2	8-17
Bitemporal hemianopia	threshold	30-2	7-18R
	threshold	30-2	7-18L
	threshold	30-2	7-19
	threshold	30-2	7-23
	threshold	30-2	7-24
Cecocentral scotoma	threshold	30-2	8-28a
Central loss, temporal wedge	threshold	30-2	8-13

MAIN FINDING	EXAMINATION TYPE	ARRAY USED	FIGURE NUMBER
Central scotoma	threshold	30-2	7-12
	threshold	30-2	8-25
	threshold	30-2	8-26
Central scotomata	threshold	30-2	8-20
	threshold	macula	8-21
Correcting lens artifact	threshold	30-2	5-14
	threshold	30-2	5-15
Diffuse depression	threshold	30-2	7-11
Diffuse depression	threshold	30-2	5-24
	threshold	30-2	5-26
	threshold	30-2	5-32
	threshold	30-2	7-10L
	threshold	30-2	8-9
Diffuse depression, correcting lens power	threshold	30-2	5-20L
	threshold	30-2	5-20R
Diffuse depression, graytone artifact	threshold	30-2	5-23
Diffuse depression, incorrect lens	threshold	30-2	5-18
Diffuse depression, incorrect lens power	threshold	30-2	5-18
Diffuse loss	threshold	30-2	7-16
Diffuse loss from incorrect correcting lens	threshold	30-2	5-21
Diffuse loss of sensitivity	threshold	30-2	6-2
Diffuse loss of sensitivity, central scotoma	threshold	30-2	8-19
Diffuse loss of sensitivity, tested without add	threshold	30-2	4-15
Disc based loss	threshold	30-2	7-2
	threshold	30-2	7-5
Double arcuate scotoma	threshold	30-2	6-13
End-stage disease	threshold	30-2	4-9
	threshold	10-2	4-11
End-stage disease, stimulus V required	threshold	30-2	4-10
End-stage loss	threshold	30-2	6-16
Enlargement of the blind spot	threshold	30-2	7-6
	threshold	30-2	8-1
	threshold	30-2	8-2
Far advanced loss	threshold	30-2	6-15
Graytone construction artifact	threshold	30-2	5-22
Hemianopia	Screening	120 point	2-9
High false negatives	threshold	30-2	5-5
High fixation loss due to incorrect fixation	threshold	30-2	5-7
High fluctuation	threshold	30-2	5-8
	threshold	30-2	5-9
	threshold	30-2	6-3
Homonymous hemianopia	screening	120 point	1-11
	screening	120 point	2-7
	screening	120 point	2-8
	screening	120 point	4-3
	screening	120 point	4-4
	screening	120 point	4-5
	threshold	30-2	4-6

MAIN FINDING	EXAMINATION TYPE	ARRAY USED	FIGURE NUMBER
	threshold	30-2	7-25
	threshold	30-2	7-26R
	threshold	30-2	7-26L
	threshold	30-2	7-27a
	threshold	30-2	7-27b
Incorrect birth date	threshold	30-2	4-13
Inferior loss	threshold	30-2	7-1a
Inferior paracentral defect, nasal step	threshold	30-2	6-7
Junctional scotoma	threshold	30-2	7-21
Lens holder artifact	threshold	30-2	4-21
	threshold	30-2	5-12
	threshold	30-2	5-13
Lid artifact	threshold	30-2	5-10
	threshold	30-2	8-10
Minimal superior loss	threshold	30-2	4-7
Nasal loss	threshold	30-2	7-10R
Nasal step	threshold	30-2	4-14
	threshold	30-2	5-19
	threshold	30-2	5-25
	threshold	30-2	5-38R
	threshold	30-2	6-8
	threshold	30-2	8-6
Nerve fiber bundle defect	threshold	30-1	2-10L
	threshold	30-2	2-10R
	threshold	merged 30-1, 30-2	2-11
	threshold	30-1	4-8
	threshold	30-2	5-38L
	threshold	30-2	6-11
	threshold	30-2	6-12R
	threshold	30-2	6-12L
	threshold	30-2	8-5
	threshold	24-2	8-8
Nerve fiber bundle defects	screening	120 point	8-7
New and progressive nerve fiber bundle defect	threshold	30-2	6-20
Nondiagnostic	screening	Armaly full field	2-6
	screening	Armaly full field	4-1
Normal exam	threshold	30-2	5-16
Paracentral defect	threshold	30-2	8-11
	threshold	10-2	8-12
Paracentral defect, nasal step	threshold	30-2	5-30
Paracentral scotoma	threshold	30-2	6-4
Peripheral constriction	threshold	30-2	7-3
	threshold	30-2	7-13
	threshold	30-2	7-30
	threshold	30-2	8-16
Peripheral loss	threshold	merged 30-2, P60-2	8-22
	threshold	30-2	8-27
Progressive diffuse loss	threshold	30-2	6-17
Progressive glaucomatous defects	threshold	30-2	6-21
Progressive glaucomatous loss, new defects	threshold	30-2	6-18
	threshold	30-2	6-23

Main Finding	Examination Type	Array Used	Figure Number
Progressive low-tension glaucoma	threshold	30-2	6-24
Progressive nasal loss	threshold	30-2	6-22
Progressive nasal loss, glaucoma change	threshold	30-2	5-36
Progressive nasal loss, overview	threshold	30-2	5-34
Progressive nerve fiber loss	threshold	30-2	6-19
Pupil effect	threshold	30-2	5-17
Pupillary effects	threshold	30-2	5-17
Quadrantanopia	threshold	30-2	7-28
	threshold	30-2	7-29
Ring scotoma	threshold	30-2	8-29
	threshold	30-2	8-30L
	threshold	30-2	8-30R
	threshold	30-2	8-31a
	threshold	30-2	8-31b
Sample STATPAC printout	threshold	30-2	5-25
Sample three-in-one printout	threshold	30-2	5-1
Temporal nerve fiber bundle defect	threshold	30-2	8-3
	threshold	30-2	8-4
Temporal wedge defects	threshold	30-2	6-10
Weak projector bulb	threshold	30-2	2-3
White scotomata, 100% false positives	threshold	30-2	5-4
White scotomata, 90% false positives	threshold	30-2	5-3
White scotomata, high false positives	threshold	30-2	5-2
Worsening then improvement	threshold	30-2	5-37

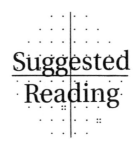

Suggested Reading

Adams AJ, Rodic R, Husted R, et al. Spectral sensitivity and color discrimination changes in glaucoma and glaucoma-suspect patients. *Invest Ophthalmol Vis Sci.* 1982; 23:516-524.

Allergan Humphrey. *STATPAC User's Guide.* San Leandro, Calif; 1987.

Anderson D. *Automated Static Perimetry.* St. Louis, Mo: Mosby; 1992.

Åsman P, Heijl A. Evaluation of methods for automated hemifield analysis in perimetry. *Arch Ophthalmol.* 1992; 110:820-826.

Åsman P, Heijl A. Glaucoma hemifield test—automated visual field evaluation. *Arch Ophthalmol.* 1992; 110:812-819.

Bebie H, Fankhauser F, Spahr J. Static perimetry: accuracy and fluctuations. *Acta Ophthalmol.* 1976; 54:339-348.

Bengtsson B, Heijl A. SITA Fast, a new rapid perimetric threshold test. Description of methods and evaluation in patients with manifest and suspect glaucoma. *Acta Ophthalmol.* In press.

Bengtsson B, Olsson J, Heijl A, RootzÄn H. A new generation of algorithms for computerized threshold perimetry, SITA. *Acta Ophthamol.* 1997; 75:368-375.

Bengtsson B, Heijl A. Evaluation of a new threshold visual field strategy, SITA, in patients with suspect and manifest glaucoma. *Acta Ophthalmol.* In press.

Bengtsson B, Heijl A, Olsson J. Evaluation of a new threshold visual field strategy, SITA, in normal subjects. *Acta Ophthalmol.* In press.

Caprioli J. Automated perimetry in glaucoma. *Am J Ophthalmol.* 1991; 111:235-239.

Caprioli J, Sears M, Miller JM. Patterns of early visual field loss in open-angle glaucoma. *Am J Ophthalmol.* 1987; 103:512-517.

Choplin NT, Sherwood MB, Spaeth GL. The effect of stimulus size on the measured threshold values in automated perimetry. *Ophthalmology.* 1990; 97(3):371-4.

Choplin NT. *Octopus Perimetry: A Meaningful Approach to Interpretation.* Huntington, WV: CILCO, Inc; 1985.

Choplin NT. Technical advances in automated perimetry: statistical analysis of visual fields. *Ophthalmic Practice.* 1992; 10(6):276-283.

deJong LAMS, Snepvangers CEJ, van den Berg TJTP, Langerhorst CT. Blue-yellow perimetry in the detection of early glaucomatous damage. *Doc Ophthalmol.* 1990; 75:303-314.

Drance SM, Anderson DR. *Automatic Perimetry in Glaucoma: A Practical Guide.* Orlando, Fla: Grune & Stratton, Inc; 1985.

Drance SM. Diffuse visual field loss in open-angle glaucoma. *Ophthalmology.* 1991; 98:1553-1538.

Duggan C, Sommer A, Auer C, and Burkhard K. Automated differential threshold perimetry for detecting glaucomatous visual field loss. *Am J Ophthalmol.* 1985, 100:420-423.

Duke-Elder S (ed). *System of Ophthalmology, Vol VII, The Foundations of Ophthalmology.* St. Louis, Mo: CV Mosby Co; 1962.Fankhauser F. Problems related to the design of automated perimeters. Doc Ophthalmol. 1979; 47:89-138.

Fankhauser F, Koch P, Roulier A. On automation of perimetry. *Albrecht v. Graefes Arch. klin. exp. Ophthal.* 1972; 184:126-150.

Fankhauser F, Spahr J, Bebie H. Some aspects of the automation of perimetry. *Surv Ophthalmol.* 1977; 22:131-141.

Felius J, de Jong LA, van den Berg TJ, Greve EL. Functional characteristics of blue-on-yellow perimetric thresholds in glaucoma. *Invest Ophthalmol Vis Sci.* 1995; 36:1665-1674.

Flammer J, Drance SM, Zulauf M. Differential light threshold: short- and long-term fluctuation in patients with glaucoma, normal controls, and patients with suspected glaucoma. *Arch Ophthalmol.* 1984;102:704-706.

Flammer J, Drance SM. Correlation between color vision scores and quantitative perimetry in suspected glaucoma. *Arch Ophthalmol.* 1984; 102:38-39.

Flammer J, Drance SM, Schulzer M. Covariates of the long-term fluctuation of the differential light threshold. *Arch Ophthalmol.* 1984;102:880-882.

Flammer J, Drance SM. Correlation between color vision scores and quantitative perimetry in suspected glaucoma. *Arch Ophthalmol.* 1984; 102:38-39.

Guthauser U, Flammer J. Quantifying visual field damage caused by cataract. *Am J Ophthalmol.* 1988; 106:480-484.

Haefliger IO, Flammer J. Fluctuation of the differential light threshold at the border of absolute scotomas—comparison between glaucomatous visual field defects and blind spots. *Ophthalmology.* 1991;98:1529-1532.

Haley MJ, ed. *The Field Analyzer Primer.* San Leandro, Calif: Allergan-Humphrey; 1987.

Hamill TR, Post RB, Johnson CA, et al. Correlation of color vision deficits and observable changes in the optic disc in a population of ocular hypertensives. *Arch Ophthalmol.* 1984; 102:1637-1639.

Harrington DO. *The Visual Fields.* 4th ed. St. Louis, Mo: Mosby; 1976.

Heijl A, Lindgren G, Olsson J. A package for the statistical analysis of visual fields. In: Seventh International Visual Field Symposium. Amsterdam; 1986.

Heijl A, Drance SM. Changes in differential threshold in patients with glaucoma during prolonged perimetry. *Br J Ophthalmol.* 1983; 67:512-516.

Herse PR. Factors influencing normal perimetric thresholds obtained using the humphrey field analyzer. *Invest Ophthalmol Vis Sci.* 1992; 33:611-617.

Heuer DK, Anderson DR, Feuer WJ, et al. The influence of decreased retinal illumination on automated perimetric threshold measurements. *Am J Ophthalmol.* 1989; 108:643-650.

Heuer DK, Anderson DR, Knighton RW, et al. The influence of simulated light scattering on automated perimetric threshold measurements. *Arch Ophthalmol.* 1988; 106:1247-1251.

Holmin C, Krakau CET. Variability of glaucomatous visual field defects in computerized perimetry. *Albrecht v. Graefes Arch. klin. exp. Ophthal.* 1979; 201:235-250.

Johnson CA, Adams AJ, Casson EJ, Brandt JD. Blue-on-yellow perimetry can predict the development of glaucomatous visual field loss. *Arch Ophthalmol.* 1993; 111:645-650.

Johnson CA. Diagnostic value of short-wavelength automated perimetry. *Current Opinion in Ophthalmology.* 1996; 7:54-58.

Johnson CA, Adams AJ, Casson EJ, et al. Progression of early glaucomatous visual field loss for blueonyellow and standard whiteonwhite automated perimetry. *Arch Ophthalmol.* 1993; 111:651-656.

Johnson CA, Adams AJ, Casson EJ, et al. Blueonyellow perimetry can predict the development of glaucomatous visual field loss. *Arch Ophthalmol.* 1993; 111:645-650.

Katz J, Sommer A. Reliability indexes of automated perimetric tests. *Arch Ophthalmol.* 1988; 106:1252-1254.

Katz J, Sommer A. Asymmetry and variation in the normal hill of vision. *Arch Ophthalmol.* 1986; 104:65-68.

Katz J, Sommer A, Gaasterland D, Anderson D. Comparison of analytic algorithms for detecting glaucomatous visual field loss. *Arch Ophthalmol.* 1991, 109:1684-1689.

Keltner JL, Johnson CA. Short-wavelength automated perimetry in neuro-ophthalmologic disorders. *Arch Ophthalmol.* 1995; 13:475-481.

Lam BL, Alward WLM, Kolder HE. Effect of cataract on automated perimetry. *Ophthalmology.* 1991; 98:1066-1070.

Lieberman MF, Drake MV. *A Simplified Guide to Computerized Perimetry.* Thorofare, NJ: SLACK Incorporated; 1992.

Lindenmuth KA, Skuta GL, Rabbani R, et al. Effects of pupillary constriction on automated perimetry in normal eyes. *Ophthalmology.* 1989; 96:1298-1301.

Lutze M, Bresnick GH. Lens-corrected visual field sensitivity and diabetes. *Invest Ophthalmol Vis Sci.* 1994; 35:649-55.

Morgan R, Feuer W, Anderson D. STATPAC 2 glaucoma change probability. *Arch Ophthalmol.* 1991; 109:1690-1692.

Olsson J, Bengtsson B, Heijl A, RootzÄn H. An improved method to estimate frequency of false positive answers in computerized perimetry. *Acta Ophthalmol.* 1997; 75:181-183.

Pokorny J, Smith VC, Verriest G, et al, eds. *Congenital and Acquired Color Vision Deficits (Current Ophthalmology Monograph).* New York, NY: Grune & Stratton, Inc; 1979.

Sample PA, Juang PSC, Weinreb RN. Shortwavelength automated perimetry for analysis of secondary and normal tension glaucoma. *Invest Ophthalmol Vis Sci (suppl).* 1994; 35:218-219.

Sample PA, Weinreb RN. Variability and sensitivity of shortwavelength color visual fields in normal and glaucoma eyes. Digest of Topical Meeting on Noninvasive Assessment of the Visual System. Washington, DC; Optical Society of America. 1993: 292-295.

Sample PA, Weinreb RN. Progressive color visual field loss in eyes with primary open angle glaucoma. *Invest Ophthalmol Vis Sci.* 1992; 33:2068-2071.

Sample PA, Weinreb RN. Color perimetry for assessment of primary open angle glaucoma. *Invest Ophthalmol Vis Sci.* 1990; 31:1869-1875.

Sample PA, Martinez GA, Weinreb RN. Color visual fields: a 5 year prospective study in eyes with primary open angle glaucoma. Perimetry Update 1991/1992: Proceedings of the Xth International Perimetric Society Meeting. Amsterdam, Netherlands: Kugler & Ghedini; 1993: 473-476.

Sample PA, Johnson CA, Haegerstrom-Portnoy G, Adams AJ. Optimum parameters for short-wavelength automated perimetry. *Journal of Glaucoma.* 1996; 5: 375-383.

Sample PA, Weinreb RN, Boynton RM. Blue-on-yellow color perimetry. *Invest Ophthalmol Vis Sci (suppl).* 1986; I27:159.

Sample PA, Taylor JD, Martinez G, et al. Short-wavelength color visual fields in glaucoma suspects at risk. *Am J Ophthalmol.* 1993; 115:225-233.

Sample PA, Weinreb RN, Boynton RM. Acquired dyschromatopsia in glaucoma. *Surv Ophthalmol.* 1986; 31:5464

Sample PA, Weinreb RN, Boynton RM. Isolating the color vision loss of primary open angle glaucoma. *Am J Ophthalmol.* 1988; 106:686-691.

Sample PA, Weinreb RN, Boynton RM. Blue-on-yellow color perimetry. *Invest Ophthalmol Vis Sci (suppl).* 1986; I27: 159.

Sample PA, Martinez GA, Weinreb RN. Short-wavelength automated perimetry without lens density testing. *Am J Ophthalmol.* 1994; 118:632-641.

Sample PA, Irak I, Martinez GA, Yamagishi N. Asymmetries in the normal short-wavelength visual field: Implications for short-wavelength automated perimetry (SWAP). *Am J Ophthalmol.* 1997; 124:46-52.

Sanabria O, Feuer WJ, Anderson DR. Pseudo-loss of fixation in automated perimetry. *Ophthalmology.* 1991; 98:76-78.

Sommer A, Enger C, Witt K. Screening for glaucomatous field loss with automated threshold perimetry. *Am J Ophthalmol.* 1987, 103:681-684.

Teesalu P, Vihanninijoki K, Airaksinen PJ, Tuulonen A, Läärä E. Correlation of blue-on-yellow visual fields with scanning confocal laser optic disc measurements. *Invest Ophthalmol Vis Sci.* 1997; 38:2452-2459.Walsh TJ, ed. *Visual Fields: Examination and Interpretation.* San Francisco, Calif: American Academy of Ophthalmology; 1990.

Werner E, Drance S. Early visual field disturbances in glaucoma. *Arch Ophthalmol.* 1977; 95:1173-1175.

Werner EB, Saheb N, Thomas D. Variability of static visual threshold responses in patients with elevated IOPs. *Arch Ophthalmol.* 1982; 100:1627-1631.

Werner EB, Adelson A, Krupin T. Effect of patient experience on the results of automated perimetry in clinically stable glaucoma patients. *Ophthalmology.* 1988; 95:764-767.

Whalen WR, Spaeth GL. *Computerized Visual Fields: What They are and How to Use Them.* Thorofare, NJ: SLACK Incorporated; 1985.

Wild JM, Moss ID. Baseline alterations in blue-on-yellow normal perimetric sensitivity. *Graefe's Arch Clin Exp Ophthalmol.* 1996; 234:141-149.

Wild JM, Moss ID, Whitaker D, O'Neill EC. The statistical interpretation of blue-on-yellow visual field loss. *Invest Ophthalmol Vis Sci.* 1995; 36:1398-1410.

Yamagishi N, Anton A, Sample PA, Zangwill L, Lopez A, Weinreb RN. Mapping structural damage of the optic disc to visual field defect in glaucoma. *Am J Ophthalmol.* 1997; 123:667-676.

Zalta AH. Lens rim artifact in automated threshold perimetry. *Ophthalmology.* 1989; 96:1302-1311.

Zangwill L, de Souza Lima M, Sample PA, Weinreb RN. Optic nerve topography in patients with short-wavelength automated perimetry visual field defects. *Invest Ophthalmol Vis Sci. (suppl).* 1996; 37:665.

Index

For your information

This book and many others on numerous different topics are available from SLACK Incorporated. For further information or a copy of our latest catalog, contact us at:

Professional Book Division
SLACK Incorporated
6900 Grove Road
Thorofare, NJ 08086 USA
Telephone: 1-609-848-1000
1-800-257-8290
Fax: 1-609-853-5991
E-mail: orders@slackinc.com
WWW: http://www.slackinc.com

We accept most major credit cards and checks or money orders in US dollars drawn on a US bank. Most orders are shipped within 72 hours.

Contact us for information on recent releases, forthcoming titles, and bestsellers. If you have a comment about this title or see a need for a new book, direct your correspondence to the Editorial Director at the above address.

*If you are an instructor, we can be reached at the address listed above or on the Internet at **educomps@slackinc.com** for specific needs.*

Thank you for your interest and we hope you found this work beneficial.